D0571795

THE FACILITATING PARTNERSHIP

THE FACILITATING PARTNERSHIP

A Winnicottian Approach for Social Workers and Other Helping Professionals

JEFFREY S. APPLEGATE, D. S. W. AND
JENNIFER M. BONOVITZ, PH.D.

JASON ARONSON INC.
Northvale, New Jersey
London

Production Editor: Judith D. Cohen

This book was set in 12 pt. New Aster by Alpha Graphics of Pittsfield, New Hampshire.

Library of Congress Cataloging-in-Publication Data
Applegate, Jeffrey S.
    The facilitating partnership : a Winnicottian approach for social workers and other helping professionals / by Jeffrey S. Applegate and Jennifer M. Bonovitz.
        p. cm.
    Includes bibliographical references (p.) and index.
    ISBN 1-56821-494-4
    1. Psychiatric social work—Methodology. 2. Winnicott, D. W. (Donald Woods) 1896–1971.   I. Bonovitz, Jennifer M.   II. Title.
    HV689.A66 1995
    362.2'0425—dc20   94-49143

Manufactured in the United States of America. Jason Aronson Inc. offers books and cassettes. For information and catalog write to Jason Aronson Inc., 230 Livingston Street, Northvale, New Jersey 07647.

Contents

PART I

WINNICOTT: PERSON, THEORIST, CLINICIAN

1

FINDING
AN APPROACH TO
HELPING

A young woman with mental retardation and a severe behavior disorder frustrates and angers the staff of her community residence with her disruptive, at times destructive actions. At her wit's end and ready to expel the client, the residence director calls in the social worker for emergency consultation. An elderly man in need of exploratory abdominal surgery refuses to leave his home—and his beloved dog— to enter the hospital for a life-saving procedure. A social worker is sent out on a home visit to intervene. A young mother receiving financial assistance brings her 3-year-old son to the hospital emergency room for treatment of a burn on his arm and is referred to social services because of suspected child abuse.

Such situations confront agency-based social workers on a daily basis. They are a sample of the kinds of problems encountered in child welfare agencies, mental health clinics, hospitals, homeless shelters, prisons, employee assistance

programs, nursing homes, drug and alcohol treatment programs, and other settings where the urgency of need and
distress seems to preclude interventions that address clients'
inner lives. Yet it may be that the vulnerable position of
needing help from another is so frightening that clients cannot easily trust and, therefore, cannot form the collaborative relationships believed to be essential for successful intervention. Feeling helpless and perplexed, social workers
may experience these untrusting clients as hard to reach,
unmotivated, or resistant. Sensing workers' frustration and
fearful of experiencing unempathic or punitive responses to
their emotional needs, these clients may act out their conflicted feelings by missing appointments or terminating precipitously. Moreover, the situations of people who appear
in many social work settings have been shaped and encum-
bered by social, political, and economic factors over which
they have little or no control. The challenge is to find an approach to helping that considers these structural and environmental factors while responding to the dynamics of the
individual client's inner experience.

Through decades of service to people in great need, social workers have developed practice-based knowledge and
skills that can be powerfully effective but are often difficult
to articulate. Terms like *support, sustainment, acceptance,*
and phrases like "environmental manipulation," "starting
where the client is," and "maintaining a non-judgmental
attitude" abound in the social work literature. These words,
the lexicon of social work practice wisdom, are intuitively
accessible but conceptually elusive. They name but do not
fully capture the nuanced complexity and dynamics of
interventions employed in professional episodes with clients.
In search of concepts and language that can give voice to
the ineffable in its work, the profession has borrowed widely
from various social and behavioral theories.

In this book we argue that the developmental and clinical theories of Donald Woods Winnicott offer a uniquely

useful set of concepts for articulating the "silent," supportive and sustaining, relationship-focused interventions that
constitute the core praxis of social work across service settings. The reader may ask—and reasonably so—why do we
need to borrow more theory from outside our professional
discipline? Don't we need to stop our promiscuous borrowing and settle down to work on explicating social work's
unique concepts and skills? And why more psychodynamic
theory? After all, our history is filled with evidence of hunt-
ing and gathering forays into psychodynamic territory. In
the late 1920s and '30s, classical Freudian drive theory informed social work practice in psychiatric hospitals, schools,
and child guidance clinics (Popple 1983). In the 1940s and
'50s, ego psychology gained popularity with social workers
because it included cultural and environmental influences
and made room for recognizing clients' conflict-free adaptive and coping capacities (Goldstein 1984, Mackey 1985).
In the 1960s, '70s, and '80s, after deinstitutionalization
moved many clients with severe disturbances out of psychiatric hospitals, social workers in community mental health
centers found object relations theory and self psychology to
be clinically useful. More recently, findings emerging from
psychoanalytically informed research on infant development
have added new conceptual ammunition to the social
worker's armamentarium.

There is a simple explanation for our propensity to borrow theory from other disciplines: we need all the help we
can get. Faced with the most perplexing and challenging of
human difficulties, we learned early in the profession's development that no one explanatory theory could encompass
the diversity of people and situations we are likely to encounter in the cluttered realities of our day-to-day practice. As a
result, we have become shrewd borrowers and creative syn-
thesizers of a variety of theories and have found innovative
ways to translate them into practice in unpredictable—indeed, sometimes overwhelming—professional episodes. We

have employed a sophisticated systems framework within which to conceptualize varying combinations of the psychodynamic "psychologies" (Pine 1988, 1990) just described. And, as needed, we have added cognitive, social learning, existential, and, more recently, narrative and other constructivist concepts to the mix. The result is more than add-and-stir eclecticism, however; it is a unique way of knowing that draws on and integrates formal theory, intuition, personal knowledge, and a century of experience on the front lines of human services.

Cohering the multiple elements of this epistemology is a focus on the helping relationship as the catalyst for change. Though social workers know what they mean by using the helping relationship in their work, they have had difficulty explicating its nuances clearly and convincingly. It is here that psychodynamic theory in general, and Winnicott's contributions in particular, become especially pertinent. His concepts offer an accessible language for spelling out the intricacies of relationship building, and they provide a way of thinking about intervention that keeps the helping relationship in the spotlight whether we are providing food and shelter or psychotherapy—or both. Moreover, many of Winnicott's formulations lend depth and precision to social work's person-in-environment perspective—a perspective that, while claimed as our identifying focus, remains conceptually elusive and difficult to apply.

Winnicott's attention to the role of the *other* in human development is the central factor that gives his formulations such compelling clinical utility (Fromm and Smith 1989; Khan 1975). From more than 60,000 consultations with infants and their caregivers (Rudnytsky 1991), Winnicott developed concepts that highlight the importance of the earliest caregiving relationship in enabling infants to begin to put the bits and pieces of their inner and outer worlds together. He then transposed these concepts to clinical work with children and adults. He recognized that, by attending to the universal relationship dynamics that are rooted in earliest interactions but reverberate throughout life, clinicians help clients put the bits and pieces of their worlds together.

Winnicott saw in infants an innate drive, referred to by Bollas (1989) as a destiny drive, to elaborate and establish the nascent true self or personal idiom. He believed, however, that this drive could be potentiated only in a facilitating partnership with caregiving others. His unique contribution lies in the detailed explication of the nuances and intricacies of this supportive relationship and their transposition to psychotherapeutic practice. The relationship-focused interventions emerging from Winnicott's work accomplish more than bolstering coping capacities, strengthening defenses, or helping the client get through the acute phase of a crisis. Our experience as clinicians and educators suggests that practice based on his ideas can also promote psychological growth. Traditional conceptions of psychodynamic psychotherapy are based on an assumption that structural change occurs primarily as the result of insight gained through the interpretation of intrapsychic conflicts and defenses as they emerge in transference to the clinician. In contrast, the post-classical view to which we subscribe contends that the internal experience evoked by the supportive and sustaining clinical relationship can also be mutative and structure-building (DeJonghe et al. 1992). This idea derives from a psychology that combines an understanding of intrapsychic conflict with an understanding of the profound impact on psychic development of early deprivation, trauma, and associated developmental arrest.

Winnicott (1954) referred to such arrest as a *"freezing of the failure situation,"* along with which "goes an unconscious assumption (which can become a conscious hope) that opportunity will occur at a later date for a renewed experience in which the failure situation will be able to be unfrozen and reexperienced, with the individual in a regressed state, in an environment that is making adequate adaptation" (p. 281, italics original). He called this regressed state a "regression to dependence" (Winnicott 1955–1956, p. 297) that, while frightening and disruptive, also offers unique opportunities for reworking early trauma and developmental conflict as well as for building psychic structure. In the interest of efficiency and cost containment, many current approaches emphasize techniques designed to avert or reverse this regression to promote rapid symptom improvement. As managed health care increasingly enters the consulting room, for example, clinicians are asked to make assessments and intervention plans quickly, often after one session, and to intervene in ways that bring rapid relief of distress. Then, in order to obtain authorization for further treatment, they are required to chart client progress in the accomplishment of specific behavioral goals—goals that may have little to do with the client's core difficulties.

This agenda, demanding a focus on outcome rather than on the therapeutic process, puts clinicians at risk of neglecting the details of relationship building and, thus, of foreclosing the emergence of dependence and its associated therapeutic potential in the treatment situation. This symptom-based approach pathologizes dependency and leaves its strengths unrecognized and untapped. The danger is that primary developmental vulnerabilities remain unaddressed and unresolved, leading clients to re-establish the maladaptive situations that replicate original deprivation and trauma. Paradoxically, in many instances fiscally driven managed health care sets up the conditions for increased expenditure as clients return for services again and again, their core psychosocial issues unseen and untreated. They remain frozen in failure.

In contrast, Winnicott saw in a person's regression to dependence an unconscious effort to return to the true self, to repair gaps in ego development, and, thus, to remobilize psychosocial growth. By welcoming and accepting the client's dependency, he offered himself as a new object—someone who was reliable, consistent, and able to withstand and survive the intensity of the client's frightening impulses and feelings. Contrasting this approach to the classical psychoanalytic stance, he noted that "Whereas in the transference neurosis the past comes into the consulting-room, in this work it is more true to say that the present goes back into the past, and *is* the past" (Winnicott 1955–1956, pp. 297–298).

When distressing current circumstances bring the traumatic past to life, feelings of helplessness and vulnerability are inevitably aroused in the helping relationship. Winnicott's approach emphasizes helping the client re-experience and begin to give voice to these feelings in a safe therapeutic environment. Here, the clinician makes friends with the client's regression to dependency, inviting it into full development. The resulting experience of relating to a new person who can tolerate and actively help with integrating the sadness, rage, and other strong affects associated with early deprivation or trauma is believed to mobilize the innate tendency toward self-reparation. Such an approach does not always require extended time, but it does require making the therapeutic relationship the primary focus, regardless of the nature of the service being provided.

Recently, in tandem with the broader application of psychoanalytic theory to people whose vulnerabilities stem from early environmental deprivation interwoven with intrapsychic conflict, clinicians of all persuasions have greeted Winnicott's ideas with renewed interest and enthusiasm. Since the mid-1980s, several new collections of his papers have appeared (see Goldman 1993a, C. Winnicott et al. 1989, D. W. Winnicott 1984, 1986b, 1988a, b, 1993) and there is a growing body of scholarship about his ideas and their clinical application (see Clancier and Kalmanovitch 1987, Davis and Wallbridge 1981, Dockar-Drysdale 1991, Fromm and Smith 1989, Giovacchini 1990, Goldman 1993a, b, Grolnick 1990, Grolnick and Barkin 1978, Phillips 1988). Scholars of psychoanalytic metapsychology have identified Winnicott as a pivotal figure in the paradigm shift in psychoanalytic theory from a drive-based to a relational psychology (Greenberg and Mitchell 1983, Hughes 1989, Rudnytsky 1991). Several social work authors have written about the particular relevance of Winnicott's concepts to their work in a variety of settings (Applegate 1984, 1989, 1990, 1993, Applegate and Barol 1989, Chescheir 1985, Chescheir and Schulz 1989, Kanter 1990, Sanville 1991, Zerbe 1990).

Our specific goal in this book is to concentrate on key Winnicottian concepts that are particularly well-suited to agency-based practice with people whose psychosocial well-being has been compromised by acute situational disruption or trauma, chronic psychological disturbance, or early environmental deprivation and related developmental vulnerabilities. We are thinking here of people who are unlikely to seek mental health services voluntarily or who do so only in periods of crisis. In various states of assimilation of their circumstances, such clients may find it difficult to reflect upon and articulate their inner experience and, therefore, do not respond readily to traditional insight-oriented psychotherapeutic approaches. Although the book's clinical examples are drawn from social work practice, human service professionals of all persuasions are increasingly encountering deprived and traumatized clients. We trust, therefore, that the book will also be useful to psychiatrists, psychologists, psychiatric nurses, case managers, and others working in a wide array of health and mental health settings, both public and private.

In the remainder of this chapter, we will introduce Winnicott. First we will provide a biographical sketch, noting some of the factors in his development that likely shaped his unique approach to clinical work and rendered it congruent with social work values, principles, and epistemology. Then we will consider Winnicott the theorist, suggesting that he was ahead of his time and would take delight in social work's current interest in constructivist ideas. A sketch of Winnicott the clinician will complete this introductory portrait and lay the groundwork for a detailed examination of his theory and its application to practice.

WINNICOTT THE PERSON

Winnicott was born in 1896 in Devon, Plymouth, England, and grew up in what his biographers describe as economically comfortable and stable circumstances. His father, John Frederick Winnicott, was 41 when Donald was born and, in addition to his work as a merchant, was active in the public life of the town, serving twice as its mayor. As was typical of British nuclear families of the time, Winnicott's father focused much of his life outside the home and apparently maintained a degree of emotional distance from its domestic center. Winnicott wrote little about his mother, Elizabeth. Recorded descriptions of her by family friends are vague and idealized, extolling her friendliness, warmth, and openness. More revealing is a poem Winnicott composed late in his life that suggests that dynamics in his relationship to her shaped his later career interests and direction.

> Mother below is weeping
> weeping
> weeping
> Thus I knew her
>
> Once, stretched out on her lap
> as now on dead tree
> I learned to make her smile
> to stem her tears
> to undo her guilt
> to cure her inward death
> To enliven her was my living.
> [quoted in Phillips 1988, p. 29]

As noted by Phillips (1988), this poem appears to embody Winnicott's recollection of "an early experience of his mother's depression, and her consequent inability to hold him" (p. 29). Phillips suggests that the poem provides clues to the origins of Winnicott's preoccupation as a theoretician with how children of depressed or withdrawn caregivers learn to put the caregiver's needs ahead of their own. He concludes that a child reared in such circumstances "might . . . have to make a living out of keeping his mother alive" (Phillips 1988, p. 30).

Certainly, although Winnicott did consider the father's role in early development (see Davis and Wallbridge 1981, pp. 133–135), he focused the spotlight of his theoretical inquiry into the deepest recesses of the child's relationship to the mother. Indeed, Winnicott's writing about this first relationship reflects an unusually intimate familiarity with the dynamics of maternal care. All three of Winnicott's recent biographers (Goldman 1993b, Phillips 1988, Rudnytsky 1991) suggest that Winnicott's family situation contributed to this capacity to identify with the feminine. His two sisters were 5 and 6 years old when he was born, and there were, in addition to his mother, a cook, a nanny, and a governess in the household. As a boy, Winnicott spent a great deal of time in the kitchen, causing his mother to complain that he spent more time with the cook than with the rest of the family. He seemed drawn to the maternal, nurturant core of the house. In autobiographical notes, Winnicott referred to himself as "in a sense . . . an only child with multiple mothers"— a child whose father apparently did little to dilute this matrifocal intensity: "it is probably true that in the early years he left me too much with all my mothers" (cited in Phillips 1988, p. 28). Whatever its origins, Winnicott's early sensitivity to the feminine and the maternal undoubtedly influenced his later theorizing.

There is biographical evidence that Winnicott's absorption in the concept of dependency and its vicissitudes also had its origins in his youth. He recalled that, after breaking his collarbone playing rugby at boarding school, "I could see that for the rest of my life I should have to depend on doctors if I damaged myself or became ill, and the only way out of this position was to become a doctor myself" (cited in Phillips 1988, p. 31). Alongside a strong feminine identification developed a determination to master dependency by becoming expert in taking care of others.

By the time he reached adolescence Winnicott knew he wanted to become a doctor and began reading medicine at Cambridge at age 18. By 1920, he was a qualified physician specializing in children's medicine. At 23 he read Freud's (1900) *The Interpretation of Dreams*, the book that introduced him to psychoanalysis. He subsequently sought training in both child and adult analysis, and over the course of his long career became an increasingly visible and outspoken figure in the British Psycho-Analytical Society, serving two terms as its president.

Winnicott's first marriage, at age 28—the same year he entered his first analysis, with James Strachey—was troubled from the beginning. Suggestions from several sources indicate that his wife suffered from a significant psychiatric disturbance that eventually led to her institutionalization and impaired the couple's relationship for its duration. Lending strength to the hypothesis that Winnicott had a need to care for troubled women is the observation that he devoted much of his young adulthood to his wife's care (Clancier and Kalmanovitch 1987). Only when he believed her to be strong enough to tolerate it did they divorce, when he was 53 years old. Though it is unclear why Winnicott never had children of his own, the strain in this marriage undoubtedly played a part. While he never spoke directly about his childlessness, a clue to the way he may have compensated for it emerges from a 1957 paper in which he notes that "people with no children can and do find all sorts of other ways of in fact having a family; they may be found sometimes to have the largest families of all" (p. 43). Perhaps the thousands of children he treated in his long career as a pediatrician and psychoanalyst comprised his "family."

Indeed, Winnicott's caregiving instincts pervaded his professional life. Through his activities in the World War II Evacuation Project and his practice in a pediatric clinic in London's poverty-stricken East End, he became acutely attuned to issues of family fragmentation, homelessness, neglect, deprivation, and other sequelae of environmental failure (Phillips 1988). This work introduced him to many social workers, one of whom, Clare Britton, became his second wife. They were apparently well matched, having many mutual interests; a friend once described them as "two crazy people who delighted each other and delighted their friends" (C. Winnicott 1989, p. 14). As professional collaborators, they practiced and wrote about what today is called mental health "case management" (Kanter 1990).

Clare Winnicott's (1989) reminiscences suggest that, as a middle-aged and older man, Winnicott was energetic, optimistic, and possessed an insatiable capacity for play—the latter a characteristic that, despite recurrent heart and lung problems, he retained until his death in 1971, at age 75. Even into old age he was given to mischievous spontaneity, exemplified by his habit of riding his bicycle with his feet on the handlebars—a practice that once prompted a policeman to stop him and exclaim, "Fancy an old man like you setting an example to everybody" (C. Winnicott, quoted in Rudnytsky 1991, p. 193). He prized playfulness as "an experience, always a creative experience . . . a basic form of living" (C. Winnicott 1989, p. 3). He enjoyed music, poetry, and dancing, and apparently made whimsical "squiggle" drawings part of his daily routine. His committment to a life fully lived is captured in a prayer found posthumously in notes for his unfinished autobiography, to be entitled "Not Less Than Everything." The prayer asks simply, "Oh God! May I be alive when I die."

WINNICOTT THE THEORIST

Winnicott's vitality spilled over into his professional and scholarly life, and he is remembered for his insistence on being himself. Indeed, as noted by Goldman (1993b), "Winnicott's personal strivings were so consistently echoed in his theoretical conceptualizations that one cannot easily disentangle his creative concepts from the person that he was" (p. 3). Masud Khan (1975), a former patient of Winnicott's and one of his key exponents, notes that "His theories are abstractions of that constant happening which was Winnicott the living person and clinician" (p. xi, cited in Goldman 1993b). Contemporaries referred to him variously as a "pixie," "a bit of a Peter Pan," and "charismatic" (Grosskurth 1986). Although retaining theoretical ties to both his major mentors, Freud and Melanie Klein, he struck out on his own, discarding or reshaping theory to suit him as he gathered clinical experience.

To the consternation of colleagues, Winnicott only inconsistently documented his debt to other theorists' ideas and failed to explore in a systematic way the divergences between his ideas and those of others (Ross 1993). He was suspicious of the overintellectualized pedantry of orthodox psychoanalytic theory, believing that it blunted therapeutic spontaneity and creativity. He preferred to work and write from instinctive and intuitive sources. Yet he was not intellectually irresponsible: he stayed abreast of the medical and scientific literature, took copious notes, and insisted on scholarly rigor (Grolnick 1990). It was his talent for generating theoretical and technical novelty from a foundation of tradition and orthodoxy that has assured the endurance of his contributions.

Winnicott's creative extensions of psychoanalytic theory were shaped by his clinical experience with infants and young children and with adults who suffered from psychosis, borderline vulnerabilities, and environmental depriva-

tion and trauma. More than the analytic neutrality and interpretive finesse suitable for work with neurotics, treatment
of these people required modification of the usual parameters of analysis and called for active, supportive interventions, including environmental modification. Indeed, Winnicott thought in systems terms and, when evaluating children,
insisted on knowing families' socioeconomic circumstances.
Sounding like a social worker, he asserted that in understanding human behavior "the unit is not the individual, the
unit is an environment-individual set-up" (Winnicott 1952,
p. 99).

In applying psychoanalytic principles to children or
to adults whose regressed psychic organization tapped the
dynamics of earliest life, Winnicott entered relatively un-
charted territory. As a result, "Winnicott's map of the mind
was not just a bland schema of ego psychology, but a vivid,
populated, liveable, emotionally authentic land that both a
patient and a therapist must indwell to enable a therapy that
reaches the guts and the bones" (Grolnick 1990, p. 10).

Reaching the "guts and bones" of people's inner lives made
it necessary for Winnicott to construct what Argyris and
Schön (1974) call "theories-of-action"—theories forged in
the immediacy and uniqueness of each clinical encounter.
As Schön (1987) might put it, Winnicott left the "high ground"
of classical psychoanalysis where therapeutic actions are
believed to be guided by empirically validated theory and
entered the "swampy lowlands" of messy, confusing difficulties that elude objectively derived solutions, challenge
existing theory, and are characterized by uncertainty, ambiguity, and unpredictability. This trend in Winnicott's work
presaged the current move from positivist to constructivist
conceptions of practice. From a constructivist perspective,
perceptions and beliefs are subjectively conceived, rooted
in meaning systems of each person's making that are experienced as reality or truth. This approach emphasizes personal or "tacit knowledge" (Polanyi 1962) that makes room

for intuition, artistry, and improvisation—dimensions of practice that elude precise verbal explication. Uncertainty, rather than a problem to be overcome, becomes an opportunity for exploration, for becoming fruitfully confused.

Winnicott seemed comfortable with ambiguity, with not knowing, and in tolerating the strong feelings aroused in his patients by their uncertainty. As a theorist, he was the quintessential constructivist: though he "knew" theory, he preferred to make theory as he went along, following directions charted by his interactions with each new patient and then retrospectively checking to see if there were theoretical precedents for what he had done. As he put it, "What happens is that I gather this and that, here and there, settle down to clinical experience, form my own theories and then, last of all, interest myself in looking to see where I stole what" (Winnicott 1945, p. 145). Not surprisingly, this approach got mixed reviews from analytic colleagues who prided themselves on the empirical rigor and technical rationality of their developing "science."

WINNICOTT THE CLINICIAN

Translated to clinical work, Winnicott's approach captures the essence of what Schön (1983) calls "reflection-in-action." Clinicians practicing in this vein attempt to establish therapeutic conditions that facilitate reflective conversations with the client. Listening for the truth of the client's narrative version of the story rather than for the objective or historical truth (Spence 1982), reflective practitioners build theory as they go. Noting this constructivist thrust in Winnicott's work, Rodman (1987) comments that "One has the sense that Winnicott did not set his sights on truth with a capital T, but on truths that would not stay still, the truth that is contained in the continuous interplay of people" (p. xxvii). Such an approach allows for—indeed thrives on—trial and error.

The lack of an imperative to be prescient permits the clinician a sense of freedom and allows for a "real" conversation or meeting with the client. Clinician and client become collaborators in investigating the puzzles in the client's life; and in the process they develop a unique culture with its own language, metaphors, and intersubjectively constructed meaning system (Saari 1986, 1991). Indeed it is in the context of this therapeutic culture that narrative truth becomes vivid and compelling and provides the possibility for recovery from past hurts.

Winnicott scholars point out that his theoretical concepts do not translate readily to technique. In fact, Winnicott disliked the idea of technique, believing that it implies adherence to a set of rules, the development of specific skills, and attempts to achieve perfection of execution. These conditions were at odds with his insistence on co-constructing each therapy anew according to its unfolding relationship dynamics. Winnicott's clinical formulations, therefore, tend to be aphoristic, opaque, and elliptical, characterized by what Argyris (1980) has called "optimal fuzziness" or useful imprecision. As he once told students before a lecture, "What you get out of me you will have to pick out of chaos" (quoted in Milner 1978, p. 37). He left it to clinicians to make their own meaning of his concepts and apply them creatively. Indeed, he never comprehensively organized his clinical concepts; rather, they are woven unevenly throughout his theoretical papers and exemplified in his own accounts of his work (Winnicott 1977, 1986a) and several by patients who were in treatment with him (Guntrip 1975, Little 1985, 1990). These accounts reveal a clinician well grounded in classical theory who was free to experiment and "play" with new ideas and intuitively derived interventions.

Winnicott brought a powerful personal presence to the clinical encounter; many who came in contact with him spoke of his "poised somatic stillness" (Khan 1975). He apparently was a natural with children, seeming to have an entrancing effect on them as he fully entered their worlds of play and fantasy. He possessed an uncanny ability to grasp quickly the essence of their concerns, a gift that is engagingly illustrated in his book, *Therapeutic Consultations in Child Psychiatry* (1971f), where we find examples of stunning clinical artistry.

Perhaps Winnicott's clinical approach is captured best in his squiggle game (see 1960c). In consultations with children, he would make an impulsive, nonrepresentational line drawing and invite the child to turn it into something. The child would add a few lines, prompting Winnicott to turn it into something else, and so on. These collaborative drawings constituted both a mode of therapeutic communication and a projective test, serving as visual records of the unfolding clinical process and as stimuli to reflective play. Similarly, as Deri (1984) notes, in Winnicottian clinical work with adults, what can be called a dialogic squiggle game is often at work. In both verbal and non-verbal interchange there is a sharing of reactive imagery that fosters the client's symbol-building capacities and establishes multi-level communication.

In his work with both children and adults, Winnicott relied more on the reparative power of the therapeutic relationship than on providing interpretations. In fact, he was suspicious of the overinterpretive methods of classical analysis and believed them to be of dubious value to people whose vulnerabilities stem from early environmental deprivation. When interpretations were in order, he stressed their trial-and-error quality: "I have always felt that an important function of the interpretation is the establishment of the limits of the analyst's understanding" (Winnicott 1963a, p. 189). He wanted to retain "some outside quality by not being quite on the mark" (1962b, p. 167), thus inviting the client to make a new "squiggle."

As noted by Khan (1975), this clinical perspective finds technical expression in what Winnicott called management. Part of the daily functioning of most social workers, management consists of the supportive qualities of the therapeutic setting, including quiet, consistency, freedom from intrusion, and a climate of acceptance and respect. The clinician abstains from interpretation and, instead, provides a "sensitive body-presence" while "letting the patient move around and just be and do what he needs to do" (p. xxvi); and, as necessary, introduces environmental resources "ranging from hospitalization to care by family and friends" (p. xxvi).

Winnicott's consistent attention to and use of the client's environment distinguished his work from that of other analysts of his time. In contrast to Klein, who focused on the intrapsychic fantasy life of infants and children, Winnicott addressed the impact on inner life of the objective external situation, thus providing us with a way to understand how this might be subjectively experienced. Moving beyond Hartmann's (1939) vague "average expectable environment" and predicting the thrust of current infancy research, he attended to the complexities of real caregivers and their real interactions with their real babies in varying physical settings. As well as a projective presence in the infant's life, the caregiver of Winnicott's theory is a real or "environment mother" with human feelings and failings—not perfect, but, hopefully, "good-enough." Transposed to clinical work, such ideas underscore the importance of the real person of the therapist and the supportive aspects of the therapeutic setting. Beyond the human environment, Winnicott took inanimate surroundings into account. With his 1953 paper on transitional objects and phenomena, he became the first psychoanalytic theorist to articulate a rigorous conceptual framework for understanding people's interactions with the inanimate world.

Winnicott's formulations repeatedly emphasize that psychic development and the environment are in continuous feedback. He rejected dualistic conceptions and developed a set of concepts based on interpsychic, open-system ideas (Grolnick 1990, Sutherland 1980).

What Winnicott captures best are the developmental and clinical dynamics of the ongoing person-environment dialectic. Paraphrasing Hegel (1807), Ogden (1989) defines dialectic as "a process in which two opposing concepts create, preserve, and negate the meaning of the other as they stand in a dynamic (ever-changing) relationship to one another" (p. 259). Winnicott focused his inquiry on the dialectic between people's experiences of psychological separateness from and merger with others. He wanted to understand how people were able to achieve a simultaneous separateness from and inextricable connectedness to the outside world.

This inquiry led him to the idea of an intermediate area or *space* in which the person-environment dialectic occurs. He called this transitional area the "potential space" (Winnicott 1971d) between inside and outside, thereby offering a spatial metaphor for visualizing the dynamic area where person and environment overlap and co-create each other. This is the "silently active containing space" (Ogden 1990, p. 180) in which clinical work occurs and wherein clinician and client can make meaning of the client's situation in all its complexity and uniqueness.

As social workers we assume the salience of all aspects of the environment in understanding and helping our clients. But in the prevailing psychoanalytic zeitgeist of Winnicott's day, such specific attention to the environment was controversial, even revolutionary. When Winnicott told his second analyst, Joan Riviere, that he intended to write a book on the environment, she warned, "You write a book on the environment and I'll turn you into a frog!" (quoted in Goldman 1993b, p. 79).

Winnicott's defiance of such warnings and his persistent attention to the setting of people's lives led to formulations that bridge the microsystemic world of the individual in the family and the larger contexts of social and cultural processes. It is his skillful balance of attention to individual psychodynamics and to larger systemic concerns that renders his concepts especially pertinent to the complex, multidetermined world of social work practice. Social workers faced by people whose vulnerabilities derive from a combination of intrapsychic, interpersonal, structural, and cultural factors find many points of convergence between Winnicott's ideas and our profession's humanitarian values, principles, and mission.

Like social workers, Winnicott was not afraid to take on the most challenging situations; he distinguished himself among analysts of his time by treating psychotic, borderline, and other severely disturbed people. He was put off neither by the depth of their regressions nor the extremes of their dependency. Nor did he believe clinical practice was confined to the consultation room. He was an advocate, public spokesman, and activist for the rights of the mentally ill, dependent children, delinquents, and other vulnerable populations. He was a vocal opponent of psychosurgery, electroconvulsive therapy, aversive behaviorism, and other procedures that he believed to be dehumanizing (C. Winnicott et al. 1989, Rodman 1987). In essence, much of Winnicott's approach to understanding and aiding others is thoroughly congruent with social work's commitment to combining "people-helping" and "society-changing." Our hope in writing this book is to acquaint readers with the formulations from his work that are especially pertinent to this dual perspective and to demonstrate how they can be applied to challenging practice situations.

PLAN OF THE BOOK

Following two chapters that further introduce Winnicott's general theory of human development and disturbance, we devote Part II, Chapters 4 through 8, to a detailed examination of five of his key concepts and their application to practice. Employing detailed case illustrations to bring theory to life, the concepts of the holding environment, ego relatedness, transitional objects and phenomena, object relating and object use, and the true and false are taken up in turn and constitute the clinical core of the book. In Part III, Chapter 9 reviews the book's key concepts from a cross-cultural perspective and considers broader implications of Winnicott's work for prevention, social policy formation, education, and knowledge-building.

2

WINNICOTT'S DEVELOPMENTAL THEORY

To set the stage for applying Winnicott's ideas to clinical social work, this chapter reviews and explicates the concepts that undergird his view of human development. Readers looking for a neatly conceived schema of developmental stages or phases will be disappointed, as will those looking for a tightly ordered sequence of developmental milestones. Winnicott (1988b) believed that "It is a highly artificial procedure, this dissection out of stages of development. In fact the human child is all the time at all stages" (p. 34). He emphasized capacities rather than positions or stages; and he allowed for a wide range of individual differences in the chronological appearance of these capacities. For example, he believed that attachments to transitional objects could develop "at about 4–6–8–12 months" (1953, p. 91); and he suggested that the beginning capacity for concern and responsibility for others developed somewhere between 6 months and 2 years of age (1963d).

Winnicott gave his developmental concepts rather simple, homespun names such as *the holding environment*, *the good-enough mother*, and *the capacity to be alone*. Derived from his vast tacit knowledge of babies and their caregivers and his extensive clinical practice with children and adults, his formulations are closer to lived experience than to objective exposition. Andre Green (1978) captures this quality aptly when he describes Winnicott's thought as "above all, a richly alive experiencing rather than an erudite schematizing" (p. 178). Winnicott pared away the jargon. Many of his published papers were originally delivered as talks to a variety of audiences ranging from colleagues at psychoanalytic meetings to gatherings of teachers, child care workers, and parents. The simplicity and informality of his language have left him vulnerable to a sentimentalized trivialization of his work that can obscure its subtle ingeniousness and originality.

Key to Winnicott's theorizing are the concepts of internalization and externalization. Like other object relations theorists, he believed that, in countless interactions with the child, the caregiver's functions are gradually internalized and become the building blocks for intrapsychic structure. The ministrations of the comforting, soothing mother, for example, gradually take shape inside the baby's object world as mental representations. Balancing this process are the equilibrating forces of externalization, in which the baby's germinal wishes, fears, moods, and mental images are projected onto outside others. These twin processes are in continuous transaction, an ongoing reciprocal oscillation between inside and outside, self and other, fantasy and reality. As noted by Grolnick (1990), this is a spiral rather than a linear process, referred to by Shor and Sanville (1978) as the "spiral dialectic" of psychosocial development.

With this helix-like image of the developmental dialectic as a backdrop, we move to a description of Winnicott's conception of the developmental process. To depict this process, he employed the metaphor of a journey from dependence to independence (1963b). He divided this journey into three broad phases—absolute dependence, relative dependence, and toward independence—which can serve as components of a framework for organizing the summary that follows. This summary is organized sequentially and describes phenomena belonging primarily to the first three years of life. Readers should keep in mind, however, that the psychosocial phenomena found in these phases remain issues for the whole life span and overlap and transact throughout development.

Because Winnicott's developmental theory evolved from his detailed observations of infants and their mothers, he developed his terms accordingly. Thus, he refers to the "good-enough mother," "mother–infant mutuality," and in other ways equates early child care with mothering. Repeatedly, however, he asserts that he excludes neither fathers nor other caregivers from his formulations and uses "mother" as a kind of shorthand to capture dimensions of the nurturing provision. Although quoted material from Winnicott's work will frequently employ the term "mother," we will use the term "caregiver" in our disquisition of his ideas. This term more accurately reflects contemporary changes in family life and addresses the realities that social workers encounter in their work with children in alternative living situations. Because the infant's primary caregivers are usually women in this culture, however, we will employ the female pronoun in referring to them.

ABSOLUTE DEPENDENCE

Winnicott once declared during a meeting of the British Psycho-Analytic Society, "There is no such thing as an infant!" Later, he elaborated on this curious exclamation: "Whenever one finds an infant one finds maternal care, and without maternal care there would be no infant" (1960d,

p. 39). A baby cannot exist as a separate entity, in other words, but only as part of a relationship. Winnicott's focus, therefore, was not on the baby and the caregiver as individuals, but on the "nursing couple" created by their interactions.

Yet he did not deny the baby's existence as an individual person: "By the end of two weeks any baby has had plenty of things happen that are entirely personal" (Winnicott 1988b, p. 29). In one of the many paradoxical statements that punctuate his work, he asserts that "the infant is at one and the same time dependent and independent" (1963b, p. 84). As Winnicott saw it, the self at birth is irreducibly private, yet requires for its complete development a mediating milieu that simultaneously protects and potentiates (Eigen 1989). Though dependent on the physical care of others at first, Winnicottian newborns are individuals with a nascent or potential sense of self ready and waiting to be brought to psychosocial life through interactions with caregiving others.

With this view, Winnicott predicted the work of Stern (1985) and other developmentalists who posit an emergent sense of self at birth. Annemarie Weil (1970), for instance, asserts that the neonate's congenital equipment determines the upper and lower limits of potential development, thus explaining why not every child responds in the same way to the same type of care. One of Winnicott's major contributions is his detailed elaboration of how the maturation of these inborn potentials may be either facilitated or impeded by early experiences within the caregiver–infant matrix, or *holding environment*.

The Holding Environment

The concept of the *holding environment* is one of Winnicott's best-known contributions to psychodynamic theory. With it, he offers not only a detailed, in-depth description of the conditions necessary for adequate psychosocial development but a metaphor for the facilitating, supportive clinical setting.

Although Winnicott emphasized the interpersonal dimensions of the holding environment, he also made room for aspects of the inanimate environment. Without naming it, he offered an ecosystems conception of the holding environment: "One can discern a series—the mother's body, the mother's arms, the parental relationship, the home, the family including cousins and near relations, the school, the locality with its police stations, the county with its laws" (Winnicott 1956b, p. 310).

Like so many of Winnicott's terms, the holding environment is intuitively accessible and seems almost naively simplistic. As he elaborated it, however, the concept is complex and contains many levels of meaning. For Winnicott, the holding environment of earliest infancy consists of fundamental caregiving activities and processes that facilitate growth and development. He termed these activities *holding*, *handling*, and *object presenting* and believed that these were accompanied by corollary developmental processes of *integration*, *personalization*, and *object relating* in infants.

Holding. According to Winnicott, reliable holding provides the psychosomatic basis in infancy for what later becomes a self-experiencing human being. Even at birth, there appears to be a "bodily pre-Ego" (Anzieu 1989), akin to the emergent sense of self described by Stern (1985), which marks each infant with a distinct individuality. Proper holding facilitates the innate drive of this nascent self toward the achievement of unit status, or *integration*. Indeed, holding begins in utero where a continuity of being in the fetus takes root in the rhythmic physiological characteristics of a healthy prenatal state. So in its earliest manifestations, the infant's individuality is shaped interactively with its environment. Toward the end of pregnancy, the mother naturally turns inward and becomes preoccupied with her own body and the baby growing inside her. During this period of *primary maternal preoccupation*, likely to last for several weeks after birth, the mother appears to transfer some of her sense of herself to the fetus. This is a positive projective identification based on the mother's preverbal memories of what it was like to be a cared-for baby herself. Through the medium of this identification, the mother prepares to be optimally attuned to her new infant after birth. Thus attuned, she can imagine what the infant feels like and needs, and so is emotionally prepared to provide for these needs in a sensitive manner. Such empathic attunement and its crucial role in both normal development and in clinical work, though first explicated by Winnicott, became central in the theorizing of Heinz Kohut (1971, 1977) and subsequent proponents of self-psychology.

Though Winnicott emphasized this preoccupation in mothers, recent research evidence suggests that fathers, too, experience a state of profound relatedness to their infants' needs. From a study of families where fathers were primary caregivers for newborns, Pruett (1983) concluded that "there appears to be a very literal 'taking in' of these babies by the fathers as a profound psychological event, metaphorically analogous to the physiologic incorporation by the mother of her growing fetus" (p. 269). Even when not primary caregivers, however, many fathers experience a strong sense of affective connectedness to their neonates. Greenberg and Morris (1974) found that the fathers they studied reported a strong sense that their infants were "theirs" immediately after birth. An awareness of unique physical features, feelings of euphoria, and increased self-esteem combined to constitute a bonding phenomenon which the authors term "engrossment" (p. 526), believed to be an innate biosocial potential in all fathers.

Although the birth process temporarily disrupts the newborn's prenatal continuity of being, attuned caregivers reestablish it as they tend to her or his basic needs for food, warmth, sleep, and contact. Here holding expands to include all that the caregivers do in their physical care of the infant, including the provision of a reliable and safe inanimate environment. The emotional climate in which physical care is provided, of course, colors everything else. Through the medium of internalization, the affective valence of physical holding is converted into the manner in which the child "holds" his or her inner life. The inner experience of the baby who is diapered, bathed, and fed silently and mechanically by a depressed, emotionally detached caregiver will likely be quite different from that of the baby who receives such care from one who actively and responsively mirrors the baby's expressions through eye contact, touches him in ways that are neither understimulating nor overstimulating, and vocalizes in affective synchrony with the baby's vocalizations.

The absence of preoccupying distress or depression assures that, through their ministrations, caregivers begin to adapt responsively to the innate integrating tendencies of their infant. It is important to emphasize this need for caregivers to do the adapting: as Winnicott (1963b) put it, "a mother and father do not produce a baby as an artist produces a picture or a potter a pot . . . The parents are dependent on the infant's inherited tendencies" (p. 85). They must begin where the baby is ready to begin, alert to signals about what he or she needs. Winnicott's views on this signaling have been refined and developed in research on temperament and its impact on the infant's experience of the environment. Greenspan (1977), for example, is using research findings to help caregivers learn to read and respond adaptively to their child's unique temperament.

At the very beginning their adaptation must be almost perfect. Holding at this stage takes account of the infant's tactile, auditory, and visual sensitivity. An optimal holding environment keeps impingements—cold bathwater, loud noises, glaring lights—to a minimum. Excessively intense affect states in caregivers—levels of anger, sadness, despair, or excitement that the infant cannot yet handle—can also be impinging. Such impingements cause the infant to react defensively; and such reactions disrupt a core sense of "going-on-being":

> If reacting to impingements is the pattern of an infant's life, then there is a serious interference with the natural tendency that exists in the infant to become an integrated unit, able to continue to have a self with a past, present, and future. With a relative absence of reactions to impingements the infant's body-functions give a good basis for the building up of a body-ego. In this way the keel is laid down for future mental health. [Winnicott 1963b, p. 86]

With adequate support from a reliable holding environment, periods of ego integration oscillate with periods of what Winnicott termed *unintegration* (1962a, p. 61). Here, the infant is able to relax, to let go in a free-floating state, able to take for granted the caregivers' reliable presence and protection and to neither react to impingement nor initiate activity. This state is believed to be a precursor of the adult capacity for relaxation and the enjoyment of reverie and solitude.

Handling. As the caregivers tend to the infant's physical needs through gentle holding, handling, touching, and stimulating, there is a unifying linkage of motor, sensory, and functional experiences. These integrative experiences help the infant feel that the self dwells in and throughout the body. Winnicott gave the term *personalization* to this coming together of psyche and soma, an aspect of which is the establishment of the skin as a boundary or limiting membrane between self and other. As part of this process, the infant's skin becomes invested with the drive to live and develop and so serves as a major psychic organizer in the service of differentiating "me" from "not-me," inside from outside (McDonald 1970). Winnicott emphasized that the sense of the self as dwelling in the body was crucial to feeling thoroughly alive and was the seat of the true self.

Object presenting. The third dimension of the early hold-ing environment has to do with the way that caregivers present the world of shared reality to the child. In the inter-actions inherent in this presentation are sown the seeds of eventual *object relating* and the dawning awareness of a reality beyond the psychosomatic self. There has been much understandable confusion about the term "object" as used in psychoanalytic theory. Critics view it as dehumanizing and inaccurate when applied to persons. In the context that Winnicott used the term and as it is employed here, it should be viewed in its particular meaning as the opposite of "sub-ject," and can hence be employed to describe persons or things outside the self that have psychological significance, meaning, and corresponding mental representations.

Winnicott frequently used the interactional dynamics of the feeding situation to explicate his concept of object pre-senting. For instance: the infant begins to feel hungry and experiences the need to eat. The sensitively attuned care-giver, responding to cues from the infant that signal hun-ger, "presents" the breast or bottle in synchronized response to these cues: "the mother places the actual breast just there where the infant is ready to create, and at the right moment" (Winnicott 1953, p. 95). In another paper (1945), he put this in a different way:

> The infant comes to the breast when excited, and ready to hallucinate something fit to be attacked. At that moment the actual nipple appears and he is able to feel it was that nipple that he hallucinated. So his ideas are enriched by details of sight, feel, smell, and next time this material is used in the hallucination. In this way he starts to build up a capacity to conjure up what is actually available. [pp. 152–153]

The hungry infant's sense, then, is that she or he creates the breast or bottle repeatedly at will, evoking an illusion of an external reality that appears to conform to inner need. By skillful object presenting the caregiver fosters a temporary illusion of omnipotence in the developing infant. The "other" in the nursing couple appears to be under the infant's magical control. The first "object" of object relations, therefore, is primarily subjectively conceived, born of a sense of omnipotence and projection. It is part of a fantasy that derives from the imaginative elaboration of bodily need and gratification. Because the outside world is being presented only in titrated doses that the infant requires and can tolerate, there is no reason at first to be aware of an objective external reality.

It is during these episodes of early care that infants periodically experience a psychological state of merger with the caregiver, what Mahler (Mahler et al. 1975) refers to as caregiver–infant symbiosis. The biorhythmic dance between infant and caregiver, if well synchronized, makes it seem as though the two are one. Yet Winnicott was well aware that even very young infants were not always in this state. His thinking predicts findings from recent infancy research (Brazelton 1982, Emde 1981, Stern 1985) that suggest that infants are capable of perceiving reality objectively during periods of quiet alertness (Wolff 1959) to the stimuli around them. As Ogden (1990) points out in his interpretation of Winnicott's thinking, early experiences of oneness with and separateness from the primary caregiver coexist in dialectical opposition. One of the fundamental paradoxes that Winnicott asks us to accept without trying to resolve is that "the infant and mother are one, and the infant and mother are two" (Ogden 1990, p. 212).

Ego Relatedness

From fantasies of merger evolves an intricate mutuality or relatedness that ultimately permits the infant to discover his or her own identity. Both during feeding and at other times of being held, infants gaze into the face of the person holding them. Winnicott (1971a) believed that the caregiver's face served as a mirror to the infant's emerging sense of self: "What does the baby see when he or she looks at the mother's face? I am suggesting that, ordinarily, what the baby sees is himself or herself. In other words the mother is looking at the baby and *what she looks like is related to what she sees there*" (p. 112, italics in original).

A contented caregiver, happy with what she sees, smiles at the gazing infant, offering a positive reflection that contributes to the infant's self-esteem and sense of value. Here is the interpersonal arena in which infants learn the nuances of facial expression and the subtleties of their own feelings, including the impact they have on others. As development proceeds, there may be less dependence on getting back an image of the self solely from the caregiver's facial expressions. Gradually, mirroring interactions extend to other family members and the society at large, and "reflecting back" continues to be a fundamental dimension of all forms of communication throughout life, including therapeutic communication.

From repeated experiences of adaptive holding, handling, and object presenting and the mirroring that accompanies them, there develops between infants and their caregivers a profound mutuality that Winnicott (1958) termed *ego relatedness*. He used this term to distinguish his concept from the classical psychoanalytic view of the ego, which he found insufficient for understanding interpersonal relationships. Freud believed that the ego's structure and functions developed primarily in relation to the management of libidinal and aggressive drives, and, although he recognized the importance of the object to the child, this was not central to his theory as it evolved. While not abandoning drive theory altogether, Winnicott saw relational needs as primary and believed that much satisfaction derived from relating in terms of the ego alone, apart from instinctual considerations (Davis and Wallbridge 1981). He referred to libido and aggression in his work but gave them subsidiary status to the "drive" toward personhood, or "unit status" (Winnicott 1960d, p. 44). Winnicott saw libido as bound up with the soothing functions of the holding environment and related to the search for connectedness. And aggression, rather than the destructive drive posited by Freud, was but one aspect of a larger force toward healthy differentiation of self from others (Fromm 1989). With these formulations, Winnicott predicted the later work of social workers Gertrude and Rubin Blanck (1979) and Jean Sanville (Sanville 1991, Shor and Sanville 1978), who reinterpret drive theory in terms of the dynamics of psychosocial union and separation.

Winnicott (1958) again employs paradox to capture the unique qualities of ego relatedness. He believed that the eventual capacity to enjoy solitude derives from repeated early experiences of being "alone" in the presence of the caregiver. Further, he asserted that "It is only when alone (that is to say, in the presence of someone) that the infant can discover his own personal life" (1958, p. 34). In the ego-supportive context of the nondemanding presence of the caregiver, the infant can enjoy periods of unintegration without anxiety. When instinctual impulses and sensations appear in this context, they can be experienced as real and truly personal, tolerably moderated by the quiet, reassuring presence of a responsive other. In time, as memory and other ego capacities evolve, the baby develops a mental representation of this presence that enables him or her to forego the actual presence of the caregiver. Thus begins the establishment of a reliable, comforting internal holding environment, the foundation of psychic structure.

Winnicott (1970c) observed that, at about 3 months of age, many nursing infants will reach up and put a finger in the caregiver's mouth, symbolically "feeding" her. He saw this early manifestation of interpersonal mutuality as a developmental milestone, a behavioral signal from the infant to the world that there is a dawning awareness of others with whom reciprocal exchange is possible. In terms of the fantasy accompanying this gesture, "The baby feeds and the baby's experience includes the idea that the mother knows what it is like to be fed" (p. 250). As Winnicott saw it, here is the first appearance of what will later become a capacity for intersubjectivity and empathy. It is also the first sign that the infant is moving from absolute dependence to relative dependence on others. Through this and other *spontaneous gestures*, the developing baby both asserts the true self and begins to imagine what it might be like to be in another's shoes. It is the task of those in the immediate holding environment to receive these gestures as indicators of healthy development and respond in ways that further affirm and reinforce them.

To summarize, during the period of absolute dependence the infant begins a process of ego integration, including a consolidation of a sense that the emerging self dwells in the body. She or he establishes a rudimentary mutuality with caregivers and, in relating to them, begins to make initial contacts with external reality. To facilitate these achievements, caregivers provide an optimal holding environment, both animate and inanimate, which is reliable and keeps to a minimum disruptive impingements on the baby's innate maturational processes. They follow the infant's lead at this stage, maintaining a nondemanding presence that allows the infant to experience and integrate a range of experiences, including both quiet and excited (instinctual) states. They present external reality in doses matched to the infant's capacity to receive and integrate it into his or her sense of omnipotence. Oscillating feelings of separateness from and union with others gradually consolidate into a capacity to be psychologically alone in the presence of another, an achievement that becomes the foundation for later intersubjectivity and empathy.

What has been described, of course, is a perfectly orchestrated scenario belonging to the utopian world of theory. In reality, it is impossible to create a holding environment free from trauma, intrusion, and impingement. Winnicott knew this and had great respect for the hardiness and resilience of infants as they withstand the inevitable vicissitudes of early development. Also, he emphasized that parents and other caregivers need not be super-human to provide an adequate facilitating environment for infant development. He insisted that most "ordinary devoted" parents cull from their own upbringing the tacit knowledge they need to do a capable job. Caregivers need be only "good enough," not perfect. Indeed, as will be seen, it is essential to ongoing development that caregivers fail. It is their mistakes, misattunements, and a graduated failure of the original near-perfect adaptation that help the infant relinquish the illusion of omnipotence and join the world of shared reality.

RELATIVE DEPENDENCE

From observing infants in an informal experimental situation that he set up in his consulting room, Winnicott (1941) noted that, at about 5 or 6 months of age, there is a marked change in their behavior. Presented with a shiny object, they start to reach for it and then hesitate, looking at the caregiver as if to get permission to go on. Should they or shouldn't they pick up the object? And what will be the consequences if they do? Winnicott saw this *period of hesitation* as the first evidence of conflictual anxiety in infants. Usually, having checked out the situation, they pick up the object and begin to play. Often this play includes pretending to feed the caregiver, and infants take delight in the caregiver's pretending to be fed. After a period of this play, the infant then drops the object, as if accidentally. Once the caregiver picks it up and returns it, the infant "drops" it again, more deliberately this time, and then repeats the interchange several times. The sequence of getting rid of the object and having it restored produces considerable enthusiasm. From observing this sequence, Winnicott concluded that the 6-month-old has become able to *play* and to understand that he has an inside and that things come from outside. From the reciprocity in this game, the infant also becomes aware that the caregiver has an inside. Here is early evidence of what will eventually become the child's capacity for a relationship between whole, distinct persons.

This phenomenon corresponds chronologically to the differentiation subphase of separation-individuation described by Mahler, Pine, and Bergman (1975). The play sequence appears to be a behavioral manifestation of what they call "hatching"—the emergence from the fantasied dual unity with the primary caregiver during which the infant appears more alert, persistent, and goal directed. Stern (1985), too, notes this shift in awareness at around 6 months, observing that infants at this point become fascinated by inanimate objects and gain proficiency in manipulating them. He believes that such changes herald the consolidation of a sense of core self and a sense of a separate, self-regulating other.

From 6 to 10 months, the frequency of periods of integration increases and mental representations of self and other become more distinct, constant, and reliable. This consolidation occurs in conjunction with increased motility, initiating what Mahler calls the early "practicing" period of development. The horizons of the world expand as the baby learns to crawl, and he or she can now leave the caregiver's lap for brief separations, checking back to make sure she is still there or returning for emotional "refueling" as necessary. The sensitive caregiver picks up and affirms these signals that the infant is becoming more self-sufficient. It is as if the infant is ready to release the caregiver from responsibility for total care. Simultaneously, the caregiver's primary preoccupation of pregnancy and early post-partum months diminishes. Having provided a nearly perfect adaptation to the young infant's needs and having participated in his or her illusion of omnipotent control of the external world, now the good-enough caregiver begins unconsciously to provide a carefully calibrated failure of adaptation. She adapts less and less perfectly, in synchrony with the infant's increased ability to deal with her inevitable failures. Busy with something else, for example, she may wait a bit longer than usual to respond to the baby's cry. Or she may introduce frustration deliberately in the form of weaning. The increasingly frequent interpersonal spaces between the infant's need and the caregiver's responsiveness heighten the infant's sense of separateness. The illusion of omnipotence gives way gradually to disillusionment, a process that is essential to further development and differentiation.

It is a fundamental assumption of psychoanalytic developmental theory, gleaned from both infant observation and from reconstructions of early experience in child and adult psychoanalysis, that experiences of gratification are experienced by the infant as pleasurable or "good" and that experiences of frustration are experienced as emotionally painful or "bad." By extension, the caregiver who responds in tandem with the infant's need and desire is "good" and loved by the infant; the one who postpones and frustrates is "bad" and hated. Internal images derived from good and bad experiences coalesce into mental representations of good and bad, loved and hated caregivers, as though the two were distinct. Further, from the mirroring experiences of mutuality described above, infants are believed to internalize mental representations of themselves that correspond to these affective polarizations. The gratified and loving infant self is "good"; the frustrated and hating infant self is "bad." At this early stage in development, the infant possesses neither the cognitive equipment nor the emotional maturity to integrate these two aspects of self and other. The two are split; hence the term *splitting* to describe the way infants organize self and object representations before the achievement of a capacity for ambivalence, or a tolerance for experiencing loving and hateful feelings toward the same person. To explain his view of how this split is mended, Winnicott proposed a process that constitutes one of his most creative and enduring contributions to psychoanalytic developmental theory.

The Transitional Process

As the previously omnipotently controlled caregiver de-adapts herself in conjunction with the infant's need to tolerate and master her inevitable failures, separation anxiety appears. The primary illusion of an omniavailable caregiver begins to falter. Because the "good" and "bad" mental representations are not yet integrated, the infant must find ways for self-soothing at times of need or distress when the caregiver's absences and other inevitable failures arouse anger and frustration. These affects must be experienced in doses that do not overwhelm the baby's capacity to handle them. The attuned caregiver prevents the baby from becoming flooded by excessive internal and external stimuli that might engender a stage of organismic distress equivalent in intensity to panic attacks seen in adults (Mahler and McDevitt 1980). In Winnicott's words, "She knows she must postpone her own impulses until the time when the child is able to use her separate existence in a positive way. She knows she must not leave her child for more minutes, hours, days than the child is able to keep the idea of her alive and friendly" (1962c, p. 71). Ultimately, the child must find a way to retain an internal image of the "good-enough" caregiver during experiences when the primary feelings toward her are "bad." To assist them in this imaginal retention, many babies reach into the nearby inanimate environment for a symbolic substitute for the caregiver.

Winnicott (1953) coined the term *transitional object* to describe the security blanket, piece of blanket, or soft, pliant stuffed animal that the baby uses to keep his or her anxiety at manageable levels. This object, whose smell, taste, and texture evoke the soothing maternal presence, is frequently taken into the mouth along with a thumb or fingers while falling asleep or at times of distress. As examples of less concrete *transitional phenomena*, Winnicott included "an infant's babbling or the way an older child goes over a repertory of songs and tunes while preparing for sleep" (1953, p. 89). He believed that transitional objects and phenomena enable infants to maintain the illusion of the gratifying caregiver while they build up a capacity to tolerate and benefit from disillusionment. Evocative of earliest feeding experiences, the transitional object can be reproduced at will to recapture the comforting illusion of the ever-available, optimally gratifying nurturer.

Implicit in this concept is a paradox that further captures the person-environment dialectic that Winnicott worked to explicate. The baby "creates" the object by imbuing it with his or her own symbolism; yet the object was there all the time, waiting to be found and created, or given symbolic meaning. There is a tacit agreement between infants and caregivers not to challenge this paradox. Good-enough caregivers proceed as though the baby had created the object and maintains control over it; but they also acknowledge its objective reality in the world of other people (Greenberg and Mitchell 1983). This tacit collusion permits the baby a chance to integrate gradually the knowledge that his or her sense of omnipotence has been illusory and that valued others are self-regulating, separate people.

Winnicott saw the transitional object as the baby's first true creative act, a bridge between the worlds of fantasy and reality (Grolnick and Barkin 1978). It exists in an *intermediate area of experiencing* between self and other, person and environment: "It is an area which is not challenged, because no claim is made on its behalf except that it shall exist as a resting-place for the individual engaged in the perpetual human task of keeping inner and outer reality separate yet inter-related" (Winnicott 1953, p. 90). From its earliest manifestations in attachments to specific objects or phenomena, a transitional process takes shape that helps people cope throughout life with the strain of reconciling inner and outer reality. The capacity to engage in the transitional process is central to a later appreciation for art, music, religious feeling, and other aspects of culture.

Play and potential space. For Winnicott (1971b), the intermediate area between self and other, fantasy and reality, is the realm of play, a phenomenon that he believed to be central to psychological health and adaptive development throughout the life span. He postulated that the preoccupied playing of children (and adults) is an elaboration of the transitional process. In play, children manipulate external reality in the service of fantasy and invest the objects and phenomena of play with symbolic meaning. Winnicott believed that play derives from the capacity to be alone in the presence of another. It implies trust in others and in the stability of the environment. The metaphor of play can be applied to the clinical situation. Freud (1914), for example, referred to the transference as "a playground . . . an intermediate region between illness and real life through which the transition from one to the other is made" (p. 154). And through a masterful exposition of theory and many evocative clinical examples, Sanville (1991) provides convincing evidence for Winnicott's assertion that psychotherapy is a structured elaboration of two people playing together.

Winnicott used the term *potential space* to capture the qualities of the intermediate area in which play develops. By this he meant the alive, creative, interactional field between objective reality and the subjectively constructed conception of this reality. In play and magic, people alter reality through the use of illusion. (Indeed, the etymological root of the word illusion is the Latin *ludere*, to play.) They act out strong feelings in the safety of the knowledge that their consequences are not real. They pretend to be others while retaining a sense of self. Fantasy and reality intertwine. Winnicott (1971d) believed that this potential space also becomes the location of culture and cultural experience, an extension of "creative living first manifested in play" (p. 100) that becomes part of larger shared meaning systems.

The transitional process, first expressed in concrete transitional phenomena and later in play and culture, is essential to perceiving self and others as distinct yet interrelated, and as permanent in time and space. Without this ability, people achieve neither the autonomy nor the interdependence so crucial to participating in the world of shared reality. Across the bridge provided by the transitional process, personal existence moves from a solipsistic world dominated by fantasies of omnipotence to a world where objective reality, though still colored by projective identification and illusion, can be perceived more objectively. How does this journey occur?

Object Relating and Object Use

To chart its course we must turn to Winnicott's (1971e) distinction between object relating and object use. He saw *object relating* as the subjective, projective mode of experiencing in which the other seems to be under the infant's omnipotent control. *Object use*, in contrast, is related to the infant's growing perception of the other as a self-regulating, separate other who is outside omnipotent control (Greenberg and Mitchell 1983). Here "use" should not be construed to mean exploitation; instead Winnicott meant that the infant develops a capacity for relating to others as external, objectively perceived persons who can serve as resources for growth rather than as projective entities.

To clarify how this transition occurs we must examine Winnicott's idiosyncratic conception of aggression and destructiveness, epitomized by his elliptical declaration that, on the journey from object relating to object usage, "the subject destroys the object" (1971e, p. 89). What does this puzzling statement mean? Perhaps more than any of his contemporaries, Winnicott explored the contribution of the aggressive drive to normal psychosocial development, tracing its manifestations at various phases of ego development. As previously noted, his conception of aggression was quite different from Freud's. While Freud made early, tentative investigations into the connections between aggression, exploratory activity, and mastery, he left this line of inquiry behind when he developed a "second" instinct theory that linked aggression primarily to destructive urges and the death instinct (Freud 1920). Winnicott picked up the thread of Freud's early ideas, viewing aggression as synonymous with motility, activity, and vitality—as an aspect of instinctual love that seeks externality and, thus, fuels self-object differentiation.

Here, Winnicott's terminology gets him into trouble by obscuring rather than clarifying his unique contribution. His language runs the risk of romanticizing aggression and destructiveness and does not fully account for the kinds of hostile, sadistic aggression seen in various forms of violent behavior. Certainly, Winnicott's theorizing in this area would have profited from later work by Parens and others who have deconstructed the concept of aggression more thoroughly. Drawing on longitudinal observations of children from birth on, Parens (1979) describes four developmental trends in aggression: nonaffective destructiveness, associated with infantile chewing and feeding activity; nondestructive assertion born of the drive to explore; hostile destructiveness, manifest in rage reactions; and pleasure-related destructiveness, expressed in teasing, taunting, and other derivatives of sadism. A somewhat different approach is taken by Stechler and Halton (1987), who distinguish between assertion and aggression, seeing each as arising from distinct biopsychosocial systems. These authors see assertion as deriving from a universal tendency to be active, to seek stimuli, to generate and carry out plans. It is typically associated with affects of joy, interest, and excitement. Aggression, in contrast, is viewed as deriving from an equally universal self-protective system that is reactive to perceived danger and is associated with affects of anger, fear, and distress.

From the perspective of this framework, what Winnicott described appears to be more associated with assertion than with aggression. But he did want to emphasize an element of true anger in his formulations. Here, Stechler and Halton's observation that assertion and aggression inevitably blur and overlap in complex interchanges with caregivers becomes relevant. There comes a point in the infant's exploratory assertions when caregivers may perceive them as aggressive and respond punitively, thus threatening the child and modeling aggressive behavior. At this juncture, assertion may be converted to the self-protective mechanism of aggression, an aspect of which Winnicott seems to be depicting in his theory.

This semantic confusion notwithstanding, Winnicott essentially sees assertion and aggression as necessary for rather than as impediments to human relatedness. He believed that they begin as part of a life force which, given an optimal amount of opposition by caregivers, is converted into energy available for the work of establishing a true and alive sense of self. From this perspective, aggression results when the baby reaches out in an impulsive and spontaneous gesture and meets benign opposition. This tolerable opposition, or resistance, on the part of caregivers helps the infant to define himself and the outside world. Ultimately, "The summation of motility experiences contributes to the individual's ability to start to exist, and out of primary identification to repudiate the shell and to become the core" (Winnicott 1950, pp. 213–214).

Drawing upon but modifying Klein's (1975) concept of the paranoid-schizoid position, Winnicott termed the earliest phase of the development of aggression and destructiveness as the period of *pre-concern* or "ruthlessness." Again, the feeding situation helps illustrate this. In hunger, the child approaches feeding in an instinctually excited state, and this somatic state has an equivalent in fantasy, including an imaginative hungry attack on the mother's body. As Winnicott hypothesized it, the infant at this stage is unconcerned as to the consequence of his or her attack and is not yet able developmentally to experience guilt. Because good and bad mental representations remain unintegrated, the infant cannot recognize that the person he or she "destroys" when excited is the same one that he or she values during quiet intervals. The way in which he or she becomes able to integrate these split representations is through fantasied destruction of the object and the object's non-retaliatory survival of this destruction. Winnicott's (1971e) own words best capture his unusual conception of this process: "The subject says to the object: 'I destroyed you,' and the object is there to receive the communication. From now on the subject says 'Hullo, object!' 'I destroyed you.' 'I love you.' 'You have value for me because of your survival of my destruction of you.' 'While I am loving you I am all the time destroying you in (unconscious) fantasy'" (p. 90).

Mahler and McDevitt's (1980) observations suggest later expressions of this process during the differentiation subphase of separation-individuation. They describe how the differentiating infant pulls at the mother's hair, ears, and nose, and strains his body away from her in order to have a better look. In these actions is found an aspect of attack—an aggressive testing of the caregiver's durability, boundaries, separateness—her externality. The caregiver accepts this exploratory behavior up to the point that it becomes truly destructive or painful, at which point she will gently redirect the baby's behavior, perhaps vocalizing firmly but soothingly in conjunction. Later the infant whose aggression is optimally frustrated in this manner will take increasing pleasure in the active use of his or her own body, pushing away from the caregiver and sliding down from her lap to explore the world beyond her body. Even later, derivatives of this "destructiveness" can be seen through the medium of older children's play. When toddlers play peek-a-boo, a derivative of earliest object usage, their experience when putting their hands over their eyes is that the object disappears, or is "destroyed" momentarily. By removing their hands, they can make the other person reappear, an event usually accompanied by delight and exhilaration. They see that the other person has survived the fantasied destruction. Each time the other person "survives," children are reassured of that person's and their own resilience and objective permanence. Further, caregivers usually affirm and applaud children's newfound capacity to use them as a vehicle for discovering externality and the constancy of others.

The second period in the development of aggression was termed the *stage of concern* by Winnicott (1954–55), akin to what Klein (1975) called the depressive position. At this point, the infant has begun to view the caregiver as separate (outside omnipotent control) and thus becomes concerned about the results of his instinctual (attacking) experience, both physical and emotional. It begins to dawn on the infant that the *object mother*—the target of ruthless impulses—is one and the same as the *environment mother*, or the person who reliably and empathically sustains the safety of the holding environment. It is this environment mother whom the infant begins to want to protect from the ruthlessness of his aggression.

Winnicott hypothesized that, with psychophysiological maturity, the infant begins to experience anxiety and guilt about destructive impulses—impulses which, at this point, include anger aroused by frustration. If he or she attacks the caregiver and in unconscious fantasy destroys her, she will be lost as a resource. The anxiety aroused by the idea of this prospective loss becomes manageable, however, as the infant becomes aware that he or she has a *contribution* to make to the environment mother. There is a growing confidence that, following expressions of aggression, there will be opportunities for reparation. Given the survival of a caregiver who does not retaliate, instinctually driven attacks will be followed by quiet periods of rapprochement. Winnicott termed this sequence the *benign circle*—a repeated experience of aggression, the caregiver's survival, and rapprochement—and emphasized the importance of the caregiver's "holding" the situation until the infant finds out that both destructive and loving impulses can be experienced simultaneously toward the same person. Gradually, through internalization of this circle, the infant learns to hold, or contain, a range of conflicting affects. This sequence, in other words, gives birth to the capacity for ambivalence, and, ultimately, to more complex intrapsychic structure. The object mother and the environment mother become integrated into one multidimensional mental representation of the other, while the aggressive, destructive self and the loving, protective, contributing self coalesce into an enduring, stable self-representation.

The early phase of pre-concern would seem to find expression in what Mahler, Pine, and Bergman (1975) call the *separation-individuation phase of practicing proper* (from 10 to 15 months of age), when the child is excitedly discovering the world with little concern about the consequences of his or her energetic omnipotence. Winnicott's description of the child's anxiety upon discovering the caregiver's separateness and accompanying concerns about anger correspond to the rapprochement subphase, lasting from 15 to 24 months of age, during which Mahler emphasizes the importance of the continuing libidinal availability of the caregiver. Research conducted after Winnicott's death suggests that fathers play a crucial role during the transition from object relating to object usage. While the child struggles to integrate ambivalence toward the primary caregiver, the father can serve as an island of non-conflictual support and nurturance (see Applegate 1987). Later, the father is a central figure in the transition from relationships that are primarily dyadic to what Winnicott termed "three-body" relationships—those that serve as the foundation for the Oedipus complex.

With the eventual development of a capacity for concern, the child becomes able to care about and be empathic toward others and to accept responsibility for the consequences of his or her behavior (Winnicott 1963c). Optimally, along with a greater capacity for social responsibility there develops a freedom of expression of instinctual life, both erotic and aggressive, that is an essential aspect of feeling thoroughly alive. This sense of a complex, rich inner life is balanced by an appreciation of the inner lives of others. There is a capacity to identify empathically with the feelings of others and to step back and perceive them objectively. Relationships become a rich interweave of feelings of connectedness with others alongside a sense of personal autonomy and clear interpersonal boundaries.

Even when development is optimal, however, there is always tension between subjective experience and objective reality, between self and other. Having begun life in a state of almost total dependence on others, we remain somewhat vulnerable to others' non-responsiveness or intrusiveness. Some residue of this vulnerability is inevitable, and there remains in each of us a private sanctum of subjective reality that is inaccessible to others. As Winnicott (1963a) put it, "At the centre of each person is an incommunicado element, and this is sacred and most worthy of preservation" (p. 187). The tension between union and autonomy gives rise to two fundamental existential trends: the urgent need to communicate and the simultaneous need not to be found, a dialectic expressed in children's games of hide and seek. For Winnicott (1963a), "The question is: how to be isolated without having to be insulated?" (p. 187). The inherent paradox in this question must remain unresolved and, indeed, contains the seeds of human uniqueness and creativity.

Language. The achievement of language in children both facilitates and complicates the developmental dialectic. Clearly, speech enables the child to communicate his or her needs, fantasies, frustrations, and thoughts to those around him or her, and therefore helps promote cognitive functioning and new, more nuanced levels of interaction that help consolidate a narrative sense of self (Zeanah et al. 1989). But Winnicott believed that language, in a curious way, leads to a loss of contact with the core pre-cognitive, psychosomatic self, an idea more recently elaborated by Stern (1985). Words cannot tap the body-connected preverbal vitality of self-experience in its most elemental and straightforward form. This way of knowing the self is, in essence, the "incommunicado element"—what Bollas (1987) refers to as the "unthought known." So while words connect us at a more sophisticated level, they simultaneously isolate us by failing to capture and convey the ineffable complexity of direct, lived experience. This inadequacy of language is the reason that Winnicott de-emphasized the role of interpretation in treatment while valuing and focusing on the curative qualities of the setting and other unspoken, supportive, and sustaining dimensions of the experience of the treatment relationship.

TOWARD INDEPENDENCE

Having developed a capacity for ambivalence and concern, and with the aid of free upright locomotion and speech, the child enters a phase that Winnicott (1963b) called "toward independence" (p. 91). Like Mahler's phrase "toward object constancy" (Mahler et al. 1975), Winnicott's implies that true independence is never achieved; nor would this be a desirable outcome. As Winnicott viewed it, the well-adapted individual balances a sense of personal privacy with a degree of interdependence with others. Now development unfolds into a continuous transaction between inner and outer reality, each enriched by the other: "In ever-widening circles of social life the child is identified with society, because local society is a sample of the self's personal world as well as being a sample of truly external phenomena" (Winnicott 1963b, p. 91). These circles expand to encompass school, peer groups, and related social contexts. With the "second individuation" of adolescence (Blos 1967), there are new opportunities to review and consolidate aspects of early development as physical maturity and socialization provide new testing grounds for autonomy and interdependence. Both friendships and intimate romantic relationships offer new opportunities for working out the balance between union and separation and their corresponding internal object relations.

Winnicott believed that a "good-enough" adulthood depends on access to early childhood phenomena, both verbal and preverbal. He asserted, for example, that it is crucial to retain the capacity for unintegration—for experiences of "letting go" into states of reverie and relaxation. Related to this capacity, but belonging more to the transitional process, is the capacity to enjoy art, music, spirituality, and other dimensions of culture that belong to the potential space between self and other, person and environment, fantasy and reality. He stressed the importance to mental health of an ability to play. Here he included an ability to play with ideas, an aspect of which is empathy. In empathy, one plays with the idea of being another while remaining fully aware that one is not.

The True and False Self

A fully developed capacity for empathy implies the existence of a solidly grounded, accessible *true self*. This true self has its origins in the infant's initial spontaneous gestures, both loving and hating, that, if welcomed and responded to in non-retaliatory ways by caregivers, lead to a sense of feeling real, alive, and grounded in the body. It implies a tolerance for and an ability to express or contain, as appropriate, the full range of affects and impulses. With a sense of a true self, the developing person can regress, play, dream, and imagine while keeping a foot planted in reality. Further, development of a true self means that a person can both enjoy solitude and can contribute to the larger social world in a variety of contexts and relationships.

Either because of lack of support or because of their own developmental vulnerabilities, some caregivers substitute their own "gestures" for their infant's and demand the infant's compliance. In reaction to such impingements, and varying with his or her own particular temperament, the infant, rather than feeling free to assert a body-connected true self, may construct a compliant *false self* that lacks spontaneity and may be overlain with an obsequious but subtly distancing veneer. Such children learn early to take care of their caregivers—to read and respond to others' needs with exquisite sensitivity while cutting themselves off from their own needs and impulses. As adults, they may appear outwardly successful and socially facile but report feeling that life has little meaning or substance.

Of course, given that each of us harbors "incommunicado" true-self elements that can never be thoroughly resonated in our interactions with others, we all display false-self elements. Winnicott (1960b) hypothesized several levels of false-self development, among which is the polite, public presentation of self that helps shape and order day-to-day social intercourse. Most people can regulate and modify, as needed, the extent to which they appropriately reveal aspects of their true and false selves to others. It is when the false-self elements dominate the presentation of self, resulting in a sense of disconnected emptiness and lack of access to psychosomatic vitality, that they become problematic. As noted and developed more thoroughly in later chapters, social conditions like poverty, discrimination, and oppression can serve to promote false-self development in whole segments of society. These conditions must be addressed at the structural and sociocultural as well as at the personal levels.

The true self, both the germinal core of development and successful development's crowning achievement, can be compromised at all phases of life. In the following chapter, we turn to an overview of Winnicott's concepts of human vulnerability and disturbance.

3

WINNICOTT'S CONCEPTS OF VULNERABILITY AND DISTURBANCE

Although Winnicott's theory of normal development paints an ideal picture, he was well aware of the ways in which adverse constitutional, psychosocial, family, and environmental conditions could mar this picture. Many people seen in social agencies emerge from environments where opportunities for "good-enough" caregiving and development have been severely compromised. Often clients' environments, both inanimate and animate, are barely intact. In many situations calling for social work intervention, fundamental questions concerning the integrity of the holding environment emerge: Is there a home? Is there food, heat, sanitation? Is there a network of persons who can offer emotional support? For people living in environments characterized primarily by deprivation, the developmental scenario outlined in the previous chapter changes dramatically.

ABSOLUTE DEPENDENCE

The Holding Environment at Risk

As noted, the mother's physical and emotional state during pregnancy becomes a central aspect of the prenatal holding environment. To provide optimal prenatal conditions, she, too, must be "held" by her own environment. In many of the marginal environments that social workers encounter, this systemic holding function cannot be taken for granted. Even when there is a home and basic necessities are in place, the environment may not provide protection from traumatic intrusion and impingement. For people living in poverty in the inner city, for example, threats to safety constitute a chronic stress.

More and more, the health and nutrition of mothers living in poverty suffer because of inadequate prenatal medical care. Many face delivery with apprehension instead of happy anticipation. Such conditions interfere with the mother's capacity to develop the primary maternal preoccupation so necessary for bonding with the fetus. The turning inward so crucial to her identification with the baby in utero may be foreclosed by the necessity for turning outward to assure her own survival. Even when the basics are in place, however, if the mother-to-be is an adolescent it is likely that her incomplete cognitive development and her emotional lability make it difficult for her to become preoccupied with the needs of another.

Further complicating a capacity for maternal preoccupation may be an addiction to alcohol and/or drugs that demands priority over the needs of the baby. The soaring numbers of infants born addicted begin life with an impingement that is likely to have life-long physical and emotional sequelae. Many infants with fetal alcohol syndrome or a physical dependence on cocaine, for example, are likely to be born prematurely. Their extended confinement to an incubator and other life-support facilities will likely compromise the processes of early bonding and attachment.

Once ready to go home, these babies are often hypersensitive to the touch that accompanies routine care. The skin ego (Anzieu 1989), rather than registering soothing sensations, may become a repository for representations of interactions that are frought with irritation or pain. Infants with this vulnerability seem inconsolable, fussy, and overstimulated. In contrast, if there is retardation due to brain damage, they are frustratingly slow to respond, appearing bland, disconnected, or tuned out. Both modes of behavior disrupt the synchrony of caregiver–infant mutuality that is the bedrock of adequate psychosocial development. Caregivers may find it difficult to identify positive aspects of themselves with such infants, who may not appear to be "good-enough." Instead of being an object for the projection of the good, valued self of the caregiver, these impaired infants may be experienced unconsciously by parents as a manifestation of the bad, damaged, or dreaded self. Burdened by these dynamics, the infant–caregiver dance of mutuality gets off on the wrong foot. In Spitz's (1963) terminology, the infant–caregiver dialogue so crucial to healthy development becomes "derailed."

Compromised Ego Relatedness

Interactions arising from such misattunements foster ego estrangement rather than ego relatedness. In place of a secure caregiver–infant attachment, attachment disturbances may arise (Bowlby 1988). In anxious resistant attachment, babies are prone to separation anxiety, tend to cling, and are tentative about exploring the world. Likewise, the primary caregiver may respond anxiously, evincing hypervigilance and overprotectiveness. In anxious avoidant attachment, the careseeking baby appears to expect rejection and tends to display a pseudo self-sufficiency and detachment. Accordingly, caregivers may hold and handle these infants mechanically and feed them without looking at their faces. An impaired connection around the first and most fundamental mode of communication—feeding—deprives both infants and caregivers. The infant loses opportunities for bonding, and the caregiver loses opportunities for experiencing her infant and herself as partners in a "real," mutually gratifying relationship. If the infant is perceived as an "unreal" or alien other, the caregiver cannot mirror his or her expressions; and without the chance to see himself or herself reflected back positively in the caregiver's eyes, the infant is left psychologically alone long before there exist internal representations that make this state tolerable (Applegate and Barol 1989). Instead of a nursing couple there are two detached entities. Rather than periods of integration punctuated by periods of unintegration, the infant's experience may be dominated by experiences of *disintegration*, or what Winnicott (1970b) referred to as *primitive agonies* or *unbearable anxieties*. In this state, infants "know what it is like to be dropped, to fall forever, or to become split into psychosomatic disunion" (p. 255), feelings that later can be managed only with psychotic defenses of depersonalization and derealization.

Such experiences interfere with the development of a cohesive body ego. The integration of psyche and soma, or the fundamental sense that the self "dwells" in the body, remains incomplete. Instead of a sense of bodily well-being there arises a primary sense of pain, deprivation, and anger (McDonald 1970). Indeed, pleasurable and painful skin sensations may fuse; pain can become libidinized, evidenced later in head-banging or other self-abusive behaviors that serve as misdirected attempts at self-soothing. Moreover, a sense of the skin as the first boundary between "me" and "not me" may fail to develop completely, impeding other basic processes of self-other differentiation. Winnicott (1988b) hypothesized that many psychosomatic illnesses in children and adults represent unconscious efforts to reconnect the psyche to the body.

Winnicott believed that, even in the absence of constitutional problems, repeated emotional trauma and impingement in the earliest months can on their own lead to unbearable anxieties and associated maladaptive defenses. If the infant and his or her caregivers are out of tune, the environment impinges in unpredictable ways that interrupt the infant's sense of going-on-being. Rather than gradually integrating predictable environmental changes in modulated doses, the infant who is subjected to traumatic impingement in unpredictable ways is caught off guard and can only react. And, for Winnicott, reacting is the antithesis of going-on-being. Repeated disruptions of personal continuity during the period of absolute dependence, when the infant's ego has not yet developed the functions that make the unpredictable predictable, result in a pattern of fragmentation of being.

Although aware of constitutional and hereditary factors in the etiology of autism, schizophrenia, and other psychoses, Winnicott concentrated on their derivatives as expressed in object relations. From his perspective, the psychosocial dynamics of these disturbances constitute an "environmental deficiency disease" (Winnicott 1949, p. 246) manifested in primitive defenses against the unbearable agonies associated with being emotionally "dropped" rather than "held." Such extreme defenses serve as a bastion of invulnerability from overwhelming affects; they assure that the feelings of fragmentation will never again be experienced. In a convoluted way, therefore, the psychological dimensions of autistic and schizophrenic adaptations represent strengths in that they protect the vulnerable self of earliest dependency. Similarly, Winnicott (1974) recognized the psychotic elements in normal persons, suggesting that the commonly encountered fear of a breakdown is a fear of original anxieties that have already been experienced and defended against. He believed that well-integrated people have access to primary process and other mental phenomena often seen in psychosis, and that such phenomena enrich the imagination and contribute to creativity. As he once quipped, "we are poor indeed if we are only sane" (Winnicott 1965a, p. 61).

Depressive States and the Manic Defense

Winnicott drew heavily on the work of Melanie Klein (1975) in his references to what today are called the mood disorders. He believed that some persons whose early inherited constitutional tendencies and environmental resources enable them to move beyond autism and schizophrenia develop depressive and manic defenses in response to early impingement. The depressive reactions that occur during the paranoid-schizoid or pre-concern period find expression in psychotic dissociation of self from environment. This form of depression implies inner feelings of emptiness and hopelessness, a giving-up on others as potential sources of nurture. Unlike later neurotic depression, which is related to guilt and mourning, this primary depression may express itself in schizoid states of detachment and deadness. Winnicott, as did Klein, viewed mania as a denial of this state, a flight from deadness into activity. Manic-depressive psychosis represents, as Winnicott saw it, a rhythmic oscillation between profound depressive states and the defense of hyperactivity.

RELATIVE DEPENDENCE

Vulnerabilities Associated with the Transitional Process

Of Winnicott's many innovative contributions to psychoanalytic theory, perhaps none has been subject to more attention and conceptual elaboration than his concent of transitional objects and phenomena. Mahler and her associates (Mahler et al. 1975) observed manifestations of the transitional process during the "hatching" subphase of separation-individuation. Tolpin (1971) related the transitional process to Kohut's (1971) concept of the mirroring self object, suggesting that transitional objects represent aspects of the infant's original attachment to an idealized, optimally soothing caregiver. Similarly, Blanck and Blanck (1979) believe that transitional objects and phenomena assist in the development of a self-soothing capacity in infants and young children. The concept of the transitional process has been applied to psychosocial development in adolescence (Applegate 1984), adulthood (Kahne 1967), and old age (Comstock 1981).

Winnicott (1953) made little mention of pathogenesis related to the transitional process, citing only fetishism, lying and stealing, obsessional rituals, and drug addiction as possible manifestations of difficulty. But subsequent theorists have associated psychological disturbance with a failure to develop attachments to transitional objects, a developmental arrest at the transitional object level, and distortions of the transitional process. Provence and Ritvo (1961) found that institutionalized babies tended not to form attachments to transitional objects. Disturbances in transitional relatedness have also been associated with autism (Fisher 1975), other psychoses (Fox 1977), and paranoia (Sugarman 1984). Many persons with borderline and narcissistic personality vulnerabilities appear unable to progress beyond the transitional level of development and may relate to other people as transitional "objects" (Arkema 1981, Fintzy 1971, Volkan 1973). The lack of a capacity to employ transitional objects for self-soothing or solace has also been implicated in amphetamine addiction (Berman 1972), eating disorders (Frankenberg 1984, Sugarman and Kurash 1982), and psychosomatic illness (Gaddini 1978).

In cultures where children are encouraged to sleep alone and other child-rearing practices foster their early independence from caregivers, the development of attachments to specific transitional objects is viewed as a sign of healthy development. Clinicians, therefore, routinely ask about children's transitional objects when taking developmental histories. Although such attachments appear less frequently in non-Western cultures (Applegate 1989), there is in healthy children some evidence that a transitional process is under way. In the absence of such evidence, there is a likelihood that a capacity to "use" objects, either animate or inanimate, for further growth is at risk. In borderline personality organization specifically, it is as though development remains arrested on the "borderline" between object relating and object use.

Vulnerabilities Associated with Object Relating and Object Use

When a compromised transitional process has made it difficult for the child to reconcile the split between "good" and "bad" self and object representations and, thus, to achieve a capacity for ambivalence, he or she is likely to remain arrested at a stage wherein he or she relates to objects primarily as subjectively conceived, projective entities. Primary caregivers are viewed in polarized ways, either as all good or all bad, in terms of the baby's "good" or "bad" internal states and their associated mental images. This polarization heightens rather than dilutes dependency feelings and tends to impede the baby's normal exploratory strivings toward independence. Without the aid of reliable transitional objects or phenomena to offer symbolic substitutes for maternal soothing, the child is left to struggle unassisted with unbearable anxieties. In place of cues that the baby is internalizing a representation of the soothing maternal presence to a sufficient degree that he can tolerate the caregiver's gradual de-adaptation, the caregiver receives signals that the baby cannot tolerate the separation implied in this de-adaptation. Depending on the baby's temperament and the degree of the caregiver's attunement, these signals of separation anxiety may take the form of behaviors that range from fearful clinging to demanding, angry protests. Caregivers may respond to this anxiety by indulging clinging behavior and becoming hypervigilant or becoming impatient and either detaching from or punishing the baby for angry manifestations of over-dependency. Whatever form these reactions take, they keep baby and caregiver locked in a dance choreographed around fearful dependency rather than releasing them for the reciprocal mutuality born of a gradual recognition and acceptance of separateness between two distinct, self-regulating, yet empathically attuned persons. The potential space between self and other is foreclosed, and the capacity for trust, play, imagination, and rich fantasy can be severely compromised.

As noted in the previous chapter, Winnicott hypothesized that the capacity to move from relating to objects as subjectively conceived projective entities to viewing them as objective but concerned resources for growth requires nonhostile aggression. In Winnicott's odd terminology, as the baby works through the transition from oneness to separateness, he tests the caregiver's durability and resilience by repeatedly "destroying" her. At first this assertion has a ruthless quality, the baby appearing totally egocentric and unable to express concern about the caregiver's responses to his or her behavior. Both the caregiver's and his or her own durability (constancy) is demonstrated by the caregiver's survival of these "attacks." But sometimes, taxing environmental conditions or personal developmental vulnerabilities—or both—make it difficult for caregivers to respond adaptively—to survive. Rather than applaud the child's aggressive thrusts toward differentiation, they experience them as personal attacks and retaliate punitively via abuse and/or neglect. And when the caregiver's own needs for nurturance and dependency override the child's entirely, caregivers can "use" the baby for stimulation or self-soothing—as a transitional object—a pattern often seen in child sexual abuse.

When caregivers retaliate rather than survive, or when they use the baby inappropriately as a target for their own poorly integrated affects and impulses, the benign circle of aggression-survival-rapprochement/reparation may become malignant, contaminating the child's capacity for empathy and concern for others. Images of the loved and hated object—and of the "good" and "bad" self—fail to coalesce into stable mental representations, and, through generalization, the world is subjectively perceived in terms of its capacity either to frustrate or gratify the child's needs. Splitting dominates internal life and object relations, and, as seen in severe borderline and narcissistic disturbances, unmanageable, frightening sexual and aggressive impulses are acted out in close relationships, transported inward through self-destructive acts, or numbed by dissociation and/or attempts at self-medication through drug use.

The anti-social tendency. In another scenario often seen by social workers, the potential to "use" others and the environment as resources for further development may become perverted into a compulsive need to exploit others and the environment in the service of maintaining some sense of control and self-cohesion. As noted previously, the developing child's experience of guilt and the accompanying wish to make reparation and contribute to others requires of the caregiver that she survive the baby's assertion/aggression without retaliating. When this does not happen, the child repeatedly tests the environment for its durability and resilience in hopes of discovering a safe environment. Often, there has been sufficient ego support for early integration to take place; but some loss or deprivation occurs that threatens this integration and impels the child to act in a way that forces the environment to "hold" him or her once again.

As Winnicott (1956b, 1984) characterized it, children's antisocial behavior compels the environment to notice their unconscious, acted-out feelings of deprivation. This behavior takes two primary forms—stealing and destructiveness. In stealing the child is not really looking for the object stolen, but rather seeks the attention of the loving caregiver he or she once had but lost. In destructiveness, the child tests the stability and resilience of the environment to see if it can stand the strain of his or her impulsive behavior. The destructive act constitutes a distress signal to society that the child needs boundaries and limits within which strong affects can be contained and safely expressed. In acting out, moreover, the child communicates to others at an experiential level what it feels like to be hurt, stolen from, and deprived.

Again finding elements of strength in disturbance, Winnicott (1967a) believed that this distress signal signifies hope—hope that, this time, the environment will not fail and the child will be able to reassert rights over what was rightfully his or hers. For Winnicott, the antisocial tendency represents an urge toward cure, an effort to reach back beyond the point of deprivation and make contact with the original good-enough caregiving environment. When this hope is not met by the environment, the defense of acting out becomes rigidified and disappointment is complete. The skill and cunning necessary for accomplishing antisocial acts provides a degree of secondary gain, and, untreated, what began as a tendency in childhood can be reinforced through peer-group culture in adolescence to become a life pattern of sociopathy. This combination of personal vulnerability and social reinforcement may result in an absence of wishes to make reparation and a lack of guilt or conscience about destructive, exploitative acts. Incarceration then becomes the only viable holding environment.

Vulnerabilities Associated with
the True and False Self

A less alloplastic defensive adaptation to early emotional dys-synchrony between infants and caregivers is the construction of a false self. In contrast to the antisocial tendency that persistently challenges the environment, the false-self adaptation is constructed around compliance to it. As explicated in Chapter 2, Winnicott (1960b) saw the true self as originating in the infant's earliest spontaneous gestures which, recognized and affirmed by caregivers, lead to a sense of feeling real. At its core is the aliveness of body tissues and the functioning of bodily systems. If things go well, the true self becomes the source of personal authenticity and creativity.

The false self develops as a protective shell around the true self when the caregiver either fails to read the child's spontaneous gestures or behaves in ways that compel the child to submerge his or her own gestures in the interest of keeping caregivers organized and psychologically afloat. Either because of a lack of support or their own developmental vulnerabilities, some caregivers are unable to sustain the infant's illusion of omnipotence. Instead, they substitute their own "gestures" and the infant, rather than asserting his or her own true self, learns to comply. This tendency to collapse inward and comply may be amplified by the child's own inherited constitutional and dispositional tendencies. Whatever its etiology, the outcome is that the caregiver's needs frequently override and foreclose those of the infant. In time, the infant subsumes his own needs to those of the caregiver and becomes overly attentive to the caregiver's needs. Such children become expert at picking up cues that others need attention and supplying it in ways that squelch their own strivings. This compliance may mask as attunement; but, in fact, the false self "lacks something, and that something is the *essential element of creative originality*" (Winnicott 1960b, p. 152, italics original).

Winnicott believed that the false self has three functions: it attends to the caregiver, it hides and protects the true self by complying with environmental demands, and it acts as a caretaker. These functions constitute a false appearance of self-sufficiency in the absence of nurture (Phillips 1988). Later, the false self may appear in what Speers and Morter (1980) refer to as overindividuation and underseparation in pseudomature children. These children remain attached to the caregiver through caretaking functions that make them appear mature; but their apparent autonomy is not based on solid ego structures. The underseparation between representations of a true, alive, spontaneous self and an attuned, responsive, yet self-regulating other forecloses the potential space. In extreme cases, the transitional process may be compromised in ways that impair the capacity for basic symbol formation.

In such instances, the false self replaces the true self and appears to be the "real" person. In less extreme circumstances, the false self protects the true self, yet acknowledges that a true, if hidden, self exists. In a sense, these variants of false self organization can be viewed as successful defenses. Both anorexia (Sacksteder 1989) and multiple personality (Smith 1989a) have been characterized as creative dissociative tactics that ensure the survival of a fragile true self. And social workers are familiar with the caretaker or rescuer false selves that clients construct in response to growing up in alcoholic or other types of troubled families where caregivers' vulnerabilities invite children to look after them.

Winnicott (1988b) also viewed overdevelopment of the intellectual function as a possible manifestation of false self organization. He believed that, in some instances, intellectualization represents a dissociation between psyche and soma that defends against uncomfortable feelings aroused by bodily based instincts and sensations. Instead of a psychological organization that remains grounded in the aliveness and dynamism of the body, the mind takes over, blunting emotional experience. This pattern has been observed in academically successful students whose intellectual overachievement masks considerable psychosocial fragility (Ogden 1976).

Winnicott did acknowledge that there are false self elements in psychological health; certainly a degree of compliance is a necessity in adaptive living. The typical adolescent, for example, tries on different personas both to hide feelings of vulnerability and to experiment with a variety of identities. In adulthood, false-self elements are part of the social facade that maintains formalized relationships with others while simultaneously acknowledging the existence of a more private and personal self (Phillips 1988). But in instances where the false self is the primary presentation even in intimate relationships, it is an expression of personality vulnerability and maladaptive defense.

TOWARD INDEPENDENCE

In Winnicott's schema, psychosis is an "environmental deficiency disease" resulting from constitutional vulnerabilities, failure of the holding environment, and derailed ego relatedness. Difficulties with the transitional process, object relating and use, and the true and false self derive from problems with relative dependence. Psychoneurosis, then, belongs to the process that Winnicott termed "toward independence." Here the object world moves from two- to three-body relationships and difficulties belong not to the vicissitudes of dyadic attachment, but to "the ambivalencies associated with the interrelationships between three 'whole' personalities" (Winnicott 1959–1964, p. 129). This configuration implies a tolerance for internal conflict and the existence of higher-level defenses, such as repression and

sublimation, that produce subjective discomfort but minimize acting out.

At this developmental level, there is a capacity to bear strong
affects without the threat of fragmentation. Unlike the depression described earlier that has to do with early traumatic loss
or deprivation, depression at this level is viewed by Winnicott
as a developmental achievement (see Winnicott 1963f). It
arises from experiences of guilt, conscience, and feelings of
concern and responsibility for others. This healthy depression, while uncomfortable, is valuable in that it makes true
mourning possible. Losses can be integrated and can promote
rather than arrest further development.

Similarly, anxiety at this level is related to conflicts about
instinctual impulses and relationships between whole persons rather than about abandonment and annihilation. Here
uncomfortable affects can be modified through verbal interchange (as in psychotherapy). Unlike the unbearable agonies
derived from early deprivation, neurotic anxieties are useful
signals of distress rather than affect states that overwhelm
the ego and can find expression only in acting out. As they
appear in neurosis, both depression and anxiety can promote
self-reflection and intersubjectivity.

Winnicott's views on neurosis were on the whole congruent with those of classical psychoanalysis, and, as such,
are more relevant to psychoanalysts than to the majority of
agency-based social workers. It is with his richly detailed
elaboration of phenomena belonging to preoedipal development that he struck his own creative course and made his
most valuable contributions to social work. In detailing the
environmental conditions for optimal early ego development, articulating the intricacies and vicissitudes of close
relationships, and explicating the processes that can contribute to ego vulnerability, he spoke in language that social
workers understand. He believed that social workers are in
a better position than analysts "to relate the individual's ego-

needs to social provision" (Winnicott 1960a, p. 160). Derived from a person-environment model, Winnicott's concepts offer a framework for dynamic, individualized, and balanced social work assessment and intervention.

WINNICOTT'S GENERAL APPROACH TO CLINICAL INTERVENTION AND ITS CONNECTION TO SOCIAL WORK PRACTICE

A key connection between Winnicott's approach and social work practice appears in his assertion that "cure at its root means care" (Winnicott 1970a, p. 112). The basis for all intervention, he believed, is the provision of a safe, ego-supportive therapeutic holding environment. For social workers, his most useful contribution is his careful, in-depth explication of supportive work. But, as illustrated in the chapters to follow, effective supportive intervention calls for more than caring and being kind.

The apparent simplicity of Winnicott's formulations, while making them approachable, also renders them vulnerable to concretizing and reification. There is danger, for example, in equating his methods with parenting; indeed, Winnicott often compared supportive work with aspects of empathically attuned infant care. As social workers have long known, misguided efforts to parent clients derive from an assumption that the original caregivers were somehow at fault and a fantasy that the clinician can correct their mistakes. At the least, such a posture leads to infantalizing the client in a way that is at odds with social work's collaborative approach and with the principle of self-determination. At worst, the reparenting posture leads to a barely disguised social control and fantasies of omnipotence on the part of the worker. Moreover, the equation between supportive work and caring implies that anyone who cares enough can be an adequate clinician. This assumption leads to a conclusion that those social workers assisting psychosocially vulnerable clients require little special knowledge or skill, a conclusion that flies in the face of the reality that supportive work is a highly complex undertaking that requires years of experience and training (Saari 1986).

Winnicott abhorred the idea of his work as a professionalized kindness, generalized empathy, or unconditional positive regard for clients (Rodman 1987). As he saw it, good-enough intervention balances gratification with frustration. As revealed in his accounts of work with antisocial children and adolescents, he believed in firm limits, including incarceration when necessary, to provide an adequate holding environment. He was one of the few analysts who dared to write about the feelings of revulsion and hatred that are inevitable in clinical work with disturbed people (Winnicott 1947).

Indeed, Winnicott believed that facilitative clinical work with clients whose development has been compromised by deprivation requires a fine-tuned sensitivity to countertransference reactions and impulses. Such clients often lack the capacity for true transference, a process that involves the ability to generate an illusion that is experienced simultaneously as real and unreal (Ogden 1990). Clients with this capacity, for example, can have strong feelings toward the clinician that are similar to feelings they had toward their parents; but they are aware that the clinician is not a parent. For clients whose capacity for illusion is not fully developed, there are times when the worker *is* the parent. Such clients unconsciously induce in the clinician feelings and behaviors consistent with their expectation of the ways parents would have felt or behaved (Horner 1979). As Bollas (1987) might put it, they can communicate the unthought known of early developmental trauma or environmental deprivation only through replication of that experience with the clinician. Responding to clients' projective identifications, social workers find themselves having to contain and integrate powerful ambivalent feelings. They may feel impelled to retaliate to clients' expressions of rage, or to become unhelpfully nurturant in response to their idealizations.

Monitoring countertransference reactions so that a consistent, reliable, and non-intrusive presence can be maintained is a perennial challenge for those working with very troubled clients. Such monitoring requires high levels of self-awareness, personal solidity, and durability. Most importantly, the clinician's consistency and reliability are essential to the client's eventual capacity to relate to him or her as a distinct, whole person. If this capacity is achieved, the client is able to imagine that the clinician is the original object and work out associated feelings while maintaining a working alliance with the "real" clinician. In the context of this alliance, even the most deprived and disturbed clients can be helped to understand unconscious dynamics and to explore the various levels of meaning their situations hold for them.

Here, Winnicott's understanding and use of interpretation becomes pertinent. He did not believe that interpretation and supportive work were incompatible. His was not the classical concept of interpretation based on the assumption that the clinician as expert can render the unconscious conscious by delivering insight. Rather, Winnicott's is a more constructivist view of interpretation; he interpreted to keep inquiry in motion rather than to sum it up. As he noted, he offered interpretations because "If I make none the patient gets the impression that I understand everything" (Winnicott 1962b, p. 167), thus foreclosing the mutual search for meaning. In this way, his view of interpretation is more akin to that of Saari (1988) and other constructivists who see it as part of the process of ongoing collaborative inquiry rather than a pivotal event in clinical work.

Moreover, interpretation for Winnicott served as much a sustaining, supportive function as an explanatory one: "A correct and well-timed interpretation . . . gives a sense of being held physically that is more real (to the non-psychotic) than if a real holding or nursing had taken place" (Winnicott 1988b, pp. 61–62). Again, the emphasis is on making a safe place for the client to become acquainted with and learn to express the true self. With interpretation, language becomes the vehicle for this process—a manifestation of what Stern and his associates refer to as the narrative sense of self that permits clinician and client to construct a story about the client's life (Zeanah et al. 1989).

In a paper addressed to social workers, Winnicott (1963e) offered several guidelines that, while intended for work with the mentally ill, seem applicable to a wide range of people and situations. These guidelines capture his emphasis on combining supportive interventions with a sensitivity to transference and countertransference. He described the worker's tasks as follows:

> You apply yourself to the case.
>
> You get to know what it feels like to be your client.
>
> You become *reliable* for the limited field of your professional responsibility.
>
> You behave yourself professionally.
>
> You concern yourself with your client's problem.
>
> You accept being in the position of a subjective object in the client's life, while at the same time you keep both your feet on your ground.
>
> You accept love, and even the in-love state, without flinching and without acting-out your response.
>
> You accept hate and meet it with strength rather than with revenge.
>
> You tolerate your client's illogicality, unreliability, suspicion, muddle, fecklessness, meanness, etc. etc., and recognize all these unpleasantnesses as symptoms of distress. (In private life these same things would make you keep at a distance.)
>
> You are not frightened, nor do you become overcome with guilt-feelings when your client goes mad, disintegrates, runs out in the street in a nightdress, attempts suicide and perhaps succeeds. If murder threatens you call in the police to

help not only yourself but also the client. In all these emergencies you recognize the client's call for help, or a cry of despair because of loss of hope of help. [p. 229]

These guidelines are simply stated, practical, and broad in scope. Rather than offering directives, they make room for flexibility and technical innovation while helping the social worker stay grounded in the solidity of the profession's values and traditions. They embody respect for clients' strengths and capacity for self-determination and a recognition that even disruptive, destructive behavior has meaning and represents a misdirected attempt at adaptation. The guidelines call on social workers to start where the client is and to be self-aware, empathic, ethical, reliable, accepting, non-judgmental, and equipped to employ environmental resources as necessary to ensure their own and their clients' well-being. Ultimately, they constitute a conceptual holding environment for psychodynamically oriented social work clinicians. In the following five chapters, we will demonstrate the implementation of these guidelines in a broad range of clinical encounters in diverse practice settings. This discussion will be structured around five of Winnicott's concepts that we believe have particular relevance for social work practice: the holding environment, ego relatedness, the transitional process, object relating and object use, and the true and false self.

PART II

PRACTICE

4

THE HOLDING ENVIRONMENT

When social workers first encounter the term *holding environment*, they experience a sense of instant recognition, a feeling of coming home. This sense of familiarity derives from their tacit knowledge, handed down through a century of accumulating practice wisdom, that one of the profession's primary roles is to create and sustain holding environments for people whose stability, safety, and continuity have been disrupted or have never been firmly established. Historically, "holding" individuals, families, groups, and communities has been the mission of many social service organizations, including the early Charity Organization Societies, the Settlement Houses, homeless shelters, child guidance clinics, and family service agencies. Today, the idea of holding expresses social work roles and functions ranging from the provision of food, clothing, housing, and other concrete services to the provision of psychotherapy. Indeed, the holding function has been described as "the essence of social work and the beginning link between Winnicott's concepts and good clinical practice" (Chescheir 1985, p. 220).

Winnicott frequently tied the concept of holding directly to social work practice. He declared that "the term 'casework' can be looked upon as a highly complex extension of the use of the word 'holding'" (1970a, p. 120). Elsewhere he wrote that "casework might be described as the professionalized aspect of this normal function of parents and local units, a 'holding' of persons and of situations, while growth tendencies are given a chance" (1961, p. 107). And in another instance he invited social workers to "think of casework as providing a human basket" (1963e, p. 227).

But Winnicott saw the provision of a stable holding environment as basic to all clinical work, including psychoanalysis. There is evidence that he occasionally held clients physically. In Margaret Little's (1990) account of her analysis with Winnicott, she describes periods of profound regression during which "he held my two hands clasped between his, almost like an umbilical cord, while I lay, often hidden beneath the blanket, silent, inert, withdrawn, in panic, rage, or tears, asleep and sometimes dreaming" (p. 44). But Winnicott primarily employed the idea of holding figuratively. He spoke of the holding dimension of verbal interventions in psychotherapy, giving the title *Holding and Interpretation* to a published account of the psychoanalysis of one of his patients (1986a). Process notes from this book convey the healing properties inherent in the client's sense of being "held" in the clinician's full attention, as demonstrated through questions, encouragement, sustaining comments, reflective remarks, and well-timed silences.

The relevance of the holding concept is especially obvious, however, when applied to supportive work, including environmental modification. Winnicott saw aspects of his work with the War Evacuation Project, with infants and their parents, with delinquent youth, and with the mentally ill as grounded in the idea of holding. In the treatment of people with major mental disturbances, he viewed hospitalization as the provision of a safe, structured, and protective holding environment (Winnicott 1963e)—a model for therapeutic communities that continues to guide practice in many analytically oriented in-patient settings (see Adler 1977, Brown 1981, Stamm 1985). In another instance, referring to residential care for children displaced by World War II, he noted that "therapy was being done in the institution, by the walls and the roof . . . by the cook, by the regularity of the arrival of food on the table, by the warm enough and perhaps warmly coloured bedspreads" (Winnicott 1970b, p. 221).

Such descriptions capture the holding activities that Winnicott referred to as "management." In contrast to the contemporary use of the term case management, burdened by images of bureaucratized impersonal care, Winnicott's ideas about management derived from his observations of the ordinary regulatory functions of everyday parenting (Kanter 1990). By management, he meant creating and sustaining facilitating environments for displaced or troubled people in the community—environments characterized by consistency, reliability, and protection from impingements from without and from within.

Minimizing external impingements requires providing as much quiet, privacy, and physical security as possible—conditions that can be difficult to establish in some social work settings. For instance, working in a general hospital may require talking at a bedside or in a waiting room where quiet and privacy are scarce. Home visits can be subject to intrusions from the comings and goings of family members and from other interruptions of everyday domestic life. Some agencies are located in neighborhoods characterized by a high incidence of crime and violence, compromising both clients' and clinicians' sense of safety. The community that "holds" the agency, in other words, cannot always protect it from potentially dangerous impingements. Worries about safety, in turn, can interfere with clinicians' and clients' capacity to develop a working relationship in an atmosphere of protection and trust.

Many aspects of holding are evident in the provision of concrete services. Often clients requiring these services are seen only once or twice, and the clinician's knowledge of community resources that can be mobilized quickly is crucial. If services are to be used successfully by clients, however, a knowledge of resources must be augmented by a way of thinking about the intervention that attends to its psychological meaning and process.

Mr. T., a 54-year-old homeless man, walked into a Travelers' Aid office asking for help. He appeared pale, gaunt, unshaven and his body odor was so pungent that, even though it was midwinter, the social worker found it necessary to sit beside an open window. From a question about what brought him to the agency, the worker learned that Mr. T. had been employed full time at a lumberyard until six months ago, and had been able to pay rent for a room. But after injuring his ankle on the job, he was laid off. Because his employer insisted that the accident resulted from Mr. T.'s own carelessness, he was refused workers' compensation. An illiterate man from the rural south, Mr. T. did not dispute this decision. Evicted from his rented room, Mr. T. was taken in by his sister, but she too asked him to leave after he began using his public assistance checks to buy alcohol. For the two months before coming to the agency he had been living on the street, panhandling and eating once a day at a shelter.

With the Christmas holidays approaching, Mr. T. reported feeling increasingly depressed. He tearfully recalled being "abandoned" at this time of year several years ago by his wife and son, after which he began drinking heavily and was arrested for drunk and disorderly behavior. In prison, he "found the Lord" and voluntarily entered an alcohol treatment program. He credited this program with helping him "pull myself up out of hell and start over." Now he felt himself sinking again, experienced feelings of hopelessness, and wished only for death. At times he stood on the subway platform and thought about jumping in front of a train.

The worker began talking with Mr. T. about the possibility of admission to a psychiatric hospital where his situation could be evaluated more thoroughly. She approached this plan gently, recognizing that, given Mr. T.'s history of what he experienced as abandonment by important women (wife, sister), he might experience the worker's referral to a hospital as another abandonment. While acknowledging his inability to survive much longer on the street, Mr. T. expressed fear of being "locked up" with "crazy" people and recounted frightening experiences with psychotic people in various shelters. The worker talked a bit about the hospital she had in mind, assuring him that he would find safety in the unit she was referring him to. She acknowledged the strength and determination that Mr. T. had mustered to pull himself together previously and expressed her optimism that, with support, he could do so again.

With this encouragement, Mr. T. decided to admit himself. Because he felt ashamed of his appearance, the worker called a nearby YMCA and arranged for him to take a shower and obtain a change of clothes and some toilet articles. After accompanying him to the hospital, the worker contacted Mr. T.'s sister, who agreed to take him back after discharge on the condition that he join an alcohol treatment program. Later the worker found a lawyer who was willing to help Mr. T. file a workman's compensation claim, a process that helped him begin to believe he could regain some control over his life and contributed to his successful hospital treatment.

In this case, the social worker helped Mr. T. gather the bits and pieces of his world together in the context of a respectful, non-judgmental, accepting relationship. She called on her knowledge of a variety of resources and made use of collateral contacts to construct the therapeutic holding environment, all the while affirming Mr. T.'s strengths and recognizing the validity of his call for help. By taking time during the interview to understand elements of Mr. T.'s history, to attend to his fears about hospitalization, and to consider possible dynamics in the relationship to her, the worker was able to help him accept the protective structure he needed to reconstitute his temporarily overwhelmed ego functions and defenses. Arrangements for "holding" after hospitalization helped keep his hope alive.

To offer a sense of continuity to clients who are likely to require services over a sustained period, a consistent meeting place is ideal. In some settings, social workers vie for a small number of offices or interviewing rooms, moving to different quarters as needed throughout the day. When we ask clients to adapt to a different office each time they come to the agency, we violate our espoused belief in the importance of the stability and continuity of the physical environment to people's well-being. More insidiously, we may unwittingly replicate clients' previous life experiences of being moved around or displaced in a seemingly random, uncaring manner. Under such conditions, protecting the potential space of clinical work becomes a formidable challenge. Stability in the physical features of the therapeutic setting is particularly important for clients whose external continuity has been disrupted repeatedly, and even small changes can be experienced as major ruptures of therapeutic going-on-being.

> A 6-year-old girl was referred to the school social worker after she began bedwetting and refusing to go to school following her family's eviction from their home. Abandoned by the father a year earlier, Lily, along with her mother and siblings, had been moving around to live for brief periods with various relatives. Lily told the worker how terrible it was not to know when the suitcase would be packed again and she would have to get used to sleeping on yet another sofa or strange floor. She drew pictures of her dream house and asked endless questions about the worker's house. Upon entering the office she invariably paused for a moment, scanning the furniture and giving especially careful scrutiny to the worker's desk, which was usually covered with

piles of books and papers. During one week between appointments with Lily, the worker caught up on her paperwork and cleared her desk of its usual clutter. When Lily next entered the office and looked at the empty desk, she burst into tears and ran into the hall, shouting "Go away and leave me forever!" Beyond verbal reassurance, she seemed convinced that the worker was packing up to move her office. Not until she pulled out books and papers to restore the desk to its familiar disarray could Lily be persuaded to return.

Agency policies and procedures can also compromise the integrity of the clinical holding environment in small but powerful ways. In a family agency in which one of the authors worked for several years, it was the policy to put intake calls through to social workers, on a rotating basis, at the time of the initial call. Workers were to take the prospective client's call and establish an appointment time immediately—even if they were in session. Often this arrangement meant listening briefly to the calling client's presenting problem and establishing whether or not the problem could be addressed by the agency. Although this policy ensured a quick response to the prospective client, thus capturing motivation and fostering initial engagement, it had the effect of impinging on the time and privacy of the client in session—and of interfering with the clinician's "primary therapeutic preoccupation" with this client's needs and concerns.

In another clinic setting it was the policy for families to be seen in a three-session evaluation by one therapist and then to be assigned to another for treatment. Although this arrangement was explained in detail in the first evaluation session, clients frequently repressed it. The impact of the change on clients was almost always adverse. As one 10-year-old boy put it, "You mean I'm not going to see you again ever? After I thought I could trust you! You probably weren't even listening to all the stuff I told you!" Especially for clients whose internal sense of continuity and capacity for trust are tenuous, interruptions of this type can be experienced as major internal discontinuities that can jeopardize subsequent efforts at engagement.

> Mrs. A., a 60-year-old woman, became very depressed after her husband died. Even though the marriage had been a stormy one, she was experiencing intense loneliness and what she described as "a big hole inside." The intake interview with an empathic male social worker went well. Mrs. A. reported immediate symptomatic relief and felt hopeful that counseling would be helpful. She was referred for ongoing treatment to a somewhat less experienced but very competent female worker. Mrs. A. was devastated by this transfer. At the outset of the first session with the new social worker Mrs. A. launched an attack on her credentials, her lack of experience, her demeanor, and her attempts to explore Mrs. A.'s strong reaction. Totally unprepared for Mrs. A.'s hostility, the social worker began to doubt her ability to be helpful. She felt intense anger and dislike for Mrs. A. and ended the session by telling her they could not work together.
>
> For Mrs. A., being "dropped" by the male intake social worker replicated the abandonment by her husband and mobilized intense rage. She reacted in turn by disparaging and rejecting the second worker, who was unable to hold the situation long enough to make use of her countertransference to understand Mrs. A.'s attack.

As exemplified by this case, attention to impingements from without must be balanced by careful attention to what Winnicott called impingements from within. Here he referred to strong affects and impulses arising inside the client that can erupt into consciousness and fracture the sense of "going-on-being." For clients whose backgrounds have been characterized by physical and/or emotional deprivation, or whose constitutional vulnerabilities have compromised the development of stable ego functions and defenses, the crises that prompt the need for clinical intervention can trigger "unbearable agonies" and associated feelings of disintegration.

The intensity of these feelings can lead to a frantic demand that action be taken instantly to change or fix the problem.

The clinician's efforts to encourage postponement of action and to promote reflection on the meaning of the problem to the client may be met with impatience and rage. It is crucial to realize that the demand that someone fix the problem instantly is in itself a defense—a style of functioning that the client has developed to keep unbearable anxieties in check. Rather than viewing such demands as resistance, we must acknowledge the client's strength and creativity in finding ways to keep helplessness, despair, and feelings of panic at manageable levels. Under the pressure of day-to-day agency life, this perspective can be difficult to maintain.

> Mrs. D., 27, came to a family service agency because of panic attacks that occurred each time her husband went away on a business trip. Her history revealed that her father had left the family for six weeks when she was 9 months old and had departed permanently when she was 5 years old. Left with a depressed and anxious mother, she had fended off her feelings of panic and despair by maintaining a fantasy that her father had never gone. She set a place for him at the dinner table each night, clung to clothing he had left behind, and insisted that nothing be rearranged in the apartment. These behaviors helped preserve her hope that he would return and that life would be the same as before his departure.
>
> In treatment she insisted that the social worker persuade her husband to change jobs so that he would no longer need to travel. Attempts to explore the meaning of this demand were met with rising panic and angry pleas that "someone" recognize how desperate she felt. When the worker gently suggested that Mrs. D.'s current feelings stemmed from events that happened when she was a young child and that she was trying to cope with them in the only way she knew, Mrs. D. covered her ears and drummed her feet on the floor in an effort to block out the words.

The opportunity for a helping relationship may mobilize frightening and potentially disorganizing feelings in clients who have been deprived or traumatized in their earlier development. When we ask clients, "How can I help?", we invite trust, self-disclosure, and a degree of closeness that can tap feelings of primary dependency and threaten fragile defenses. Feelings of longing and wishes to be cared for that are generated by offers of help may evoke echoes of the loss, abandonment, and deprivation that characterized earlier relationships with inconsistent caregivers. Often these feelings are globally-experienced, undifferentiated affects that, rather than being consciously recalled, have become part of the "unthought known" of pre-verbal development (Bollas 1987). Eluding words, they can be captured and communicated only through the language of action.

Unable to articulate the nuances of these feelings, clients unconsciously try to set up conditions designed to test the sincerity and durability of the clinician—to find out, as Winnicott put it, "if you may be able to prove sensitive and reliable or whether you have it in you to repeat the traumatic experiences of their past" (1963e, p. 227). In fact, the only way some clients have of communicating their internal experience is through setting up the interpersonal conditions with the clinician that replicate the dynamics of earlier primary relationships. Specifically, some clients may appear sullen, disconnected, preoccupied, openly hostile, or they may storm out of the office, fail to appear for appointments, and in other ways attempt to give the worker an experience of what other close relationships have been like for them. Through projective identification and acting out, in other words, they attempt to give the clinician an experience of being on the receiving end of disinterest, anger, or abandonment and to provoke behavior that replicates that of earlier objects.

The unconscious agenda for provoking the clinician into angry, retaliatory behaviors is twofold: it is intended to reproduce the affective experience of anxious attachment to an earlier object who, although possibly rejecting and angry, was a source of familiarity and continuity for the client; and it serves to keep the worker at a distance, thus protecting the client from regressive longings that might emerge during positive interactions. If clinicians can hold or "contain" (Bion 1962) their reactions to these provocations and reflect on their own boredom, irritation, and feelings of rejection as possible replications of aspects of the client's internal life, they may find that they are receiving valuable communications about the client's object world. Resulting empathic attunement assists the clinician to bring the client's communication into the verbal realm rather than reacting in retaliatory ways that confirm the client's expectations.

Ms. G., a 31-year-old teacher, sought help at a mental health clinic because of her inability to end a twelve-year relationship with a boyfriend who was, in her experience, either attentive and loving or preoccupied and distant. When he was loving, Ms. G. became restless and felt she should look for someone else. When he was distant she engaged his attention by threatening to leave him. On occasions when she did break off the relationship, she would become panicky, could neither sleep nor eat, and felt suicidal.

Soon after therapy began, Ms. G. began to complain that the social worker was "nice" but unhelpful and spoke about finding someone else to work with. At other times she would praise the worker effusively for her warmth and sensitivity. She began to cancel appointments at the last minute, alleging "emergencies" with the children she taught; then she would become furious when the worker was unable to accommodate her requests for evening or Saturday appointments. Soon she had created an unpredictable series of comings and goings that left the worker feeling confused, angry, and helpless. Surmising that her feelings might be mirroring aspects of Ms. G.'s internal affective state, the worker began to ask her about stories or memories of her early life that might relate to unpredictable comings and goings. Apparently just after Ms. G.'s birth, her mother became depressed and began drinking heavily. She lost interest in her infant and at times forgot to feed or change her. A concerned, loving aunt visited daily and tended to Ms. G.'s needs, but she had to return to her own family each evening. The worker concluded that Ms. G.'s internal world was dominated by contradictory images of loving and abandoning, "coming and going" objects. Because these images derived from earliest life, Ms. G. had no words to express their meaning. Rather, she "told" the worker in the only way she could—by setting up interpersonal conditions that would compel the worker to feel what she had felt. Clearly, this same form of communication governed the relationship with her boyfriend, whose intolerance for sustained closeness replicated her experiences with earlier objects.

A clinician who survives the client's testing behavior and makes a non-retaliatory, reflective response that is at odds with the client's unconscious agenda is likely to surprise him or her, potentiating a complex set of reactions. One reaction may be for the client to feel, "Here is someone different from what I've come to expect; perhaps she really does care and can help." Balancing this positive reaction, however, may be a fearful one: "Here is someone different; the unfamiliarity of her response frightens me and leaves me feeling anchorless and abandoned." Clearly the clinician must temper his or her interventions sensitively so as to "hold" the beginning relationship while affording the client as much control as possible over the parameters of closeness and distance. The ideal is to remain supportive while not becoming too confining. For some clients, meeting in any room or office is too confining and threatening to the fragile sense of self.

Doris, age 16, brought her 20-month-old daughter, Keisha, to a pediatric walk-in clinic for treatment of a lingering cold. As had happened on Doris's previous visits to the clinic, the pediatrician who saw Keisha believed that her recurring illnesses and developmental delays reflected some misattunement in the mother–daughter relationship and referred Doris to social services for help with parenting. Doris had yet to see a social worker, however. When referred on a previous occasion, she left before the worker was free to see her; and, another time when a nurse accompanied Doris to the worker's office, she excused herself to use the bathroom and did not return.

The worker realized that the first task of engagement was a pragmatic one—that of keeping Doris from fleeing. After a brief interchange in which Doris became angry and agitated, Keisha began to fuss and cry. Doris declared, "If I don't get her out of here she's going to be really evil on the bus!" Surmising that Doris was also expressing her own need to get away, the worker responded, "You both look like you're ready to leave. Why don't I walk you to the bus? I can carry the diaper bag." Doris looked suspicious: "You ain't got nothing better to do with your time? Is this what they pay you for?" Smiling in response, the worker replied, "It sounds like you're telling me that being with you and Keisha is a waste of time—as though you're not important."

As the bus pulled up, Doris agreed to another appointment; but she did not appear for it. When reached by telephone, she admitted that she didn't really want to come to the worker's office. Doing so made her feel "cooped up." She asked if she could meet the worker in the hospital cafeteria after Keisha's next clinic visit. In the interim, the worker caught sight of Doris at the bus stop and went over to say hello. As they chatted, Doris revealed more about her situation, including her considerable resentment of Keisha's father, who rejected them both when she was born. When the bus came, the worker helped Doris lift up the stroller and remarked that she was glad to see her again. Doris replied, "I'm surprised you came over after how evil I was last time."

All subsequent sessions with Doris took place either in the hospital cafeteria, the clinic waiting room, or at the bus stop near the hospital. They were successful, nevertheless, in supporting Doris in keeping regular clinic appointments for Keisha and in helping her follow through with a referral to an infant stimulation program in the community. Throughout, the worker saw Doris's behavior as neither resistance nor manipulation but as an effort to define tolerable boundaries of the holding environment. The worker's survival of Doris's "evilness" and the acceptance of her definition of the unconventional "potential space" for intervention made further work possible.

Attention to the holding environment of treatment, while crucial in initial engagement, remains important at all phases of intervention. Clinicians often fail to appreciate that such mundane modifications as changes in appointment times, absences due to illness or vacation, or the move to a different office can feel extremely disruptive to clients' sense of "going-on-being" in the treatment context. Verbal, reflective, psychologically-minded clients may be consciously or pre-consciously aware of the meaning of such changes and can process it in dialogue with the clinician. For clients whose vulnerabilities stem from preverbal periods or from profound trauma, however, even small alterations of the framework of treatment may present major disruptions to internal continuity. A planned vacation, although announced well in advance by the clinician, can feel like an abandonment; a change in offices can trigger feelings of disorientation. For many clients, these affects remain unconscious and find expression only in acting out or in projective identification. Hence, a client informed of a clinician's upcoming vacation several weeks in advance may "forget" or cancel the next appointment, thus "abandoning" the clinician as a way of letting him or her know what it feels like to be left behind. Or a client whose life has become more stable may precipitate a crisis that is intended, unconsciously, to compel the clinician to forfeit the vacation and continue the treatment without interruption. For such clients, arranging for interim coverage or offering specific information about the clinician's planned whereabouts may help dispel fantasies of abandonment.

ASSESSING THE INTEGRITY OF THE HOLDING ENVIRONMENT

Once some degree of initial engagement with the client or family has been established, assessment of the strengths and vulnerabilities in the client's past and present holding environment can proceed. Comprehensive assessment includes consideration of the degree of intactness of the client's *physical*, *interpersonal*, and *intrapsychic* holding environment. In all three of these dimensions, the clinician considers the degree to which elements in the client's environment are either facilitating or unsupportive of the client's well-being.

The Physical Dimension

Especially in work with low-income clients or those in a major crisis, careful assessment of available physical resources is primary. This process proceeds in an obvious direction. Is there housing, sufficient food, adequate clothing? Are living conditions, including the neighborhood, safe? Are they sanitary? Overcrowded? Are there environmental stressors—noise, severe pollution, dangerous social conditions—impinging on the client's situation? In gathering information about these factors, the social worker can enhance relationship-building by trying to assess the meaning of various environmental conditions to the client. What does it feel like to be in them? What do present living circumstances recall about earlier life circumstances? Are they familiar and, though perhaps objectionable from the clinician's point of view, comforting to the client?

> Mr. J. lived in public housing for the elderly. His tiny apartment was cluttered with stacks of newspapers, old cereal boxes, and odd assortments of string. In answer to a social worker's inquiry about whether he might be more comfortable and have more room to maneuver his walker if these collections were re-

moved, Mr. J. declared, "Hell, no! It's taken me years to get all this stuff together. Who knows when I'll need it? You take it away and I'll have to start over!"

Often in social work we encounter clients whose lives have been disrupted in fundamental ways but who are reluctant to accept assistance. In working with people who are homeless, for example, shelters may be available; but it is well known that many homeless people prefer living on the streets to living in shelters where they fear robbery, assault, or other dangers. Again, careful attention to the unique meaning of physical conditions and resources to individual clients should be a central focus.

> A volunteer in a church-based program for homeless families noted that Mrs. W. spent much of her time in her room and was reluctant to join the other women and children for meals. When asked why this was so, Mrs. W. burst into tears. She said that she had been a nurse and until recently had lived in her own home in a comfortable middle-class neighborhood. A fire had destroyed her house and belongings, and a subsequent lengthy illness had wiped out her life savings. She could not believe that she was now in the position of living in a shelter; she felt as though she had lost her identity and become a statistic. When the coordinator of the program had given her a newspaper with suitable job opportunities already circled in red ink, she felt devastated: "Just because I lost my home doesn't mean I've lost my capacity to think for myself!"

Conditions that may appear facilitating to helping professionals may feel like impingements to clients. Failure to try to assess the dimension of meaning may lead to a reluctance or refusal to use the resources proffered.

> In the aftermath of a large inner-city fire, the local community health center set up satellite offices to offer concrete services and counseling to families who had lost their homes. To

the surprise of administrators of this emergency program, very few families applied for help. Most of the victims of the fire were African American and tended to distrust the primarily white mental health staff. Many equated receiving concrete services with being given welfare "handouts." In this working-class community where people prided theselves on their ability to support their families, such support was unwelcome.

The Interpersonal Dimension

In tandem with determining the integrity in the client's physical holding environment, it is imperative to assess the interpersonal context. Who are key figures in the client's life? Is there a spouse or partner? Children? Extended family? Friends? Work associates? To what extent are these people facilitating or impinging on the client's well-being? Are the relationships supportive and nurturing, or are they abusive? More broadly, does the client live in circumstances wherein he or she finds compatibility and affirmation in terms of his or her race, ethnicity, culture, social class, or sexual orientation? If the client is a member of a minority group, to what extent do discrimination and oppression disrupt his or her sense of personal continuity? Each client will, of course, experience the interpersonal world in unique, idiosyncratic ways. Reflective inquiry about the meaning of various people to the client must be an aspect of comprehensive assessment.

Such inquiry is important to understanding the client's relationships to people in the past as well as to those in the present. To the extent possible, information about past relationships is best gathered over time as the client feels safe and comfortable in revealing it. Efforts to take a history or probe too intrusively for sensitive information very early in contacts with the fragile client may frighten him or her into flight from treatment or into defensive obfuscation of potentially important information.

A 35-year-old woman whose mother had been repeatedly hospitalized for manic-depressive illness during the client's childhood described her family life in idealized terms. When the social worker pressed her for details about how she felt when her mother disappeared for months at a time and left her to take care of the household, the client became agitated and angry: "You're trying to make me say things that are not true!" She failed to show up for her next appointment and did not return follow-up phone calls.

Clients whose protective defenses have led to repression or denial of aspects of early relationships may also feel inadequate when asked to recount details of growing up, thus reinforcing rather than reducing feelings of failure and poor self-esteem. For other clients, the structure offered by detailed history-taking can feel helpful. Individualization is, of course, the key to responsive assessment, and must include a consideration of developmental factors along with others.

Many clients can reflect on the meaning of their significant early relationships and the impact of these on their present lives. For those whose development has been compromised by early deprivation or trauma, however, early experiences with others may remain part of the "unthought known" (Bollas 1987). This is a dimension of internal life which, because it has neither been structured into mental representations nor found form in language, remains a "thing-of-action" rather than an "object of contemplation" (Werner and Kaplan 1963). As such, the client may be able to "tell" the clinician about his or her inner experience of others only through projective identification. In such instances, the clinician's attunement to his or her own countertransference feelings is crucial; they give important clues as to what the client is experiencing intrapsychically but cannot "think" or tell in words. Sensitivity to countertransference phenomena is helpful not just during initial assessment but throughout intervention.

Mr. R., a 36-year-old physician's assistant, came to a mental health clinic for help with marital problems and depression. He was bright, insightful, and extremely articulate. One day he came to his session and, as usual, began talking immediately. Although the content of what he said was unremarkable, even boring, the social worker began to find herself feeling increasingly uncomfortable. She could not follow what the client was saying and became acutely anxious. Mr. R. talked nonstop about one idea after another and evinced no noticeable anxiety. Puzzled by her own sense of inner disorganization, the social worker interrupted Mr. R. to ask him how he was feeling. "Oh," he replied, "I'm feeling just terrible!" He went on to say that all day he had been feeling "disconnected, like I'm in pieces scattered all over the place."

When the social worker carefully explored with him when he had first noticed this sensation, he traced it back to that morning. He had been working in the emergency room and had assisted a doctor by holding a 7-month-old baby who was undergoing a spinal tap. Mr. R. had never done this before and felt very anxious. The baby had screamed in terror when Mr. R. took her from her mother and at that point he felt himself "break up inside and just go to pieces." He did not know how he got through the procedure and had no recollection of the next hour or so. The social worker then reminded Mr. R. that he had been hospitalized at 6 months of age for evaluation of a transient seizure disorder. As she spoke, Mr. R. began to tremble and reported feelings of rising panic. His mouth became dry and his speech so thick that the social worker had to get him water before they could continue.

The Intrapsychic Dimension

The silent dialectic between the client's projective identifications and the clinician's countertransference constitutes part of the language through which assessment of the client's intrapsychic life is accomplished. Other information about this dimension emerges in gathering information about the physical and interpersonal aspects of the client's situation.

In making an assessment of the intrapsychic holding environment, the clinician can conceptualize his or her task in
terms of examining the degree to which the client experiences impingements from within. Pine's (1990) four psychologies of psychodynamic theory—those of drive, ego,
object, and self—provide a helpful organizing framework to
guide this task.

First, what is the client's degree of comfort with his or her
biologically based instinctual life, those "lasting urges . . .
forged in the crucible of early bodily and family experience"
(Pine 1990, p. 33)? Here the focus falls especially on the
wishes, conflicts, and defenses associated with sexual and
aggressive drives and impulses. Does the client manage these
drives in a modulated and satisfying manner, or do they
"manage" him or her, leading to impulse-ridden sexual and
aggressive behavior? Management of drives and impulses
is an aspect of ego-functioning and defense, the second area
of intrapsychic assessment. To what extent are primary
autonomous ego functions such as memory, perception, and
mobility operational? What about those of secondary
autonomy, such as reality testing, judgment, regulation of
affect, and the capacity to postpone gratification? What level
of cognitive functioning predominates—has formal operational thought been achieved or is the client's thinking dominated by concrete operations? Are defenses such as denial,
repression, regression, displacement, sublimation, projection, and projective identification employed flexibly according to changing but tolerable levels of anxiety, or are they
employed in a compulsive, rigid manner in order to manage a constant threat of overwhelming anxiety?

Jimmy, age 10, had been placed in foster care the day after
his fourth birthday. His father's whereabouts were unknown
and his mother was crack-addicted. She visited sporadically,
usually when she was high and unable to stay attuned to Jimmy's
feelings. Jimmy was referred to the child guidance center for

treatment when he was about to be ejected from his fourth foster home and his third elementary school. He denied having any
problems and said that it was always the other children at school
or at home who picked on him and got him into trouble.

When the social worker observed Jimmy's classroom, she
noted that he did well as long as there was activity. However,
when the teacher gave assignments that required silent concentration, Jimmy would first stare out the window and then begin to fidgit. Soon he would be nudging the child nearest him
or flicking pieces of paper around the room. Inevitably he would
be sent to the principal's office. This behavior suggested to
school personnel and to the worker the likelihood of a neuro-
logically based attention deficit hyperactivity disorder; but she
suspected that complicated psychodynamics also played a part.

His most troubling behavior at home occurred at bedtime or
when the other foster children were quietly doing homework.
The foster mother mused, "It's like he can't stand for things to
be peaceful. He always has to be in there stirring things up."
Soon this behavior appeared in interviews with the social worker.
Jimmy was in control of his behavior as long as he was racing
toy cars around the room or flying paper airplanes. As soon as
there was a lull and the social worker began inviting him to talk
about his feelings, his behavior changed dramatically. In a matter of seconds Jimmy would be knocking over a chair, kicking
a lamp, or pulling leaves off a plant. At these times he could
not respond to verbal limit-setting but required physical holding while the social worker spoke quietly, suggesting that there
were upsetting feelings that were hard to put into words.

Eventually he was able to say that when he sat quietly he
began to get a "creepy crawly" feeling. It was especially hard
for him at bedtime; the only way he could control this sensation and get to sleep was to rock back and forth vigorously—to
the extreme annoyance of his foster brother. His motoric activity both relieved his anxiety and put the distress he experienced into those around him. When it got out of bounds at
home, he was removed from his room; at school, he was sent
to the principal's office. Both the foster parents and his teachers felt angry, frustrated, and helpless. Unwittingly, they were
caught up in repetitions of a sequence of events that had oc-

curred with his mother. Desperately trying to engage her, he would behave annoyingly until in exasperation she would send him outside or to his room. When his persistent demands continued to escalate, she ultimately requested foster placement, thus sending him away forever. Jimmy's cognitive and verbal capacities were insufficiently developed to enable him to communicate the enormity of this trauma with words. He resorted to action language and the defense of projective identification, putting his feelings onto others as an eloquent but growth-inhibiting way of telling his story.

In assessing the capacity for object relations, part of the emphasis is on the extent to which the client is able to engage in mutually gratifying relationships with others. More complex is the assessment of the degree to which these relationships are ruled and distorted by internalized self and object representations forged in earliest relationships with the client's caregivers and subsequently generalized to others. Have past relationships prepared the client for experiences of trust and comfort with others, or are current relationships, including that with the clinician, colored by expectations of lack of interest, betrayal, or abandonment—of being "dropped"? While transference is ubiquitous in relationships, early deprivation or trauma can set the stage for persistent negative transferences that impede the helping process.

Finally, comprehensive assessment of the intrapsychic dimension of the holding environment requires attending to the client's sense of self, defined by Pine (1990) as the "ongoing subjective state which itself comes to have motive power in individual function" (p. 37). Winnicott's concept of "going-on-being" captures the essence of this internal state, the innermost core of which he believed to be the true self. Does the client appear to have a sense of a distinct identity that remains consistent across a variety of situations and relationships? Or is the self a chameleon-like false self that changes according to changing circumstances? Is there a feeling of cohesion about the client's sense of self, or does it appear fragmented and at the mercy of inner urges? Can the client preserve a sense of him- or herself as a distinct, self-regulating person during intimate interactions with others or does the sense of self become blurred or lost at these times? Is there a capacity to use the self as a resource, as in self-soothing, or must the client turn to external sources such as other people, objects, or mind-altering substances to sustain self-esteem and self-cohesion?

The Developmental Perspective

In assessment of the integrity of all these dimensions of the client's holding environment, it is important to keep in mind that holding is not a static concept. During various stages of psychic development needs change, and what constitutes growth-promoting holding at one stage may be experienced as impinging at another. For example, caregivers who are accustomed to physically caressing and stimulating their children in infancy will need to shift gears as the children become toddlers and enter the oedipal phase, when needs for autonomy and the establishment of appropriate inter-generational boundaries become paramount. As illustrated in the following vignette, adolescence is a time when the entire family may have to realign its holding functions to accommodate changing circumstances.

> Lynnette, 13, was referred to the school social worker after her grades began to drop and she complained of being lonely and of having few friends. Her parents noted that she had always been a quiet child who shared little about her feelings. She had been achieving well in school until sixth grade when her parents separated. At that time she began spending long periods of time in her room watching television, and her grades went from an A to a C average. Although she appeared angry and sad, she would talk with neither of her parents about her feelings.

In the first few sessions with the social worker, Lynnette expressed only anger and humiliation about having to come for help. Expressions of anger were followed by long silences during which she would stare at the floor and twiddle her hair. When the worker's efforts to help Lynnette talk continued to fail, she decided to stop pressuring her and rather attend to and comment about her nonverbal communications. She noted that Lynnette frequently brought a piece of string to the sessions, abjectly twisting it in her fingers. The worker remarked that it seemed as though Lynnette were trying to show in this behavior how knotted up she was feeling. She mused that it might be hard for Lynnette to understand and disentangle her reactions to her parents' separation. While such interventions seemed to make little impact in the sessions, Lynnette's mother reported that Lynnette had begun to tell her how angry she felt that she was seeing another man and periodically blamed her for causing her father to leave.

A few sessions later Lynnette wore a new ring whose design depicted a broken heart. She twisted it around her finger in a way that the worker was sure to notice. The worker commented that she thought Lynnette was trying to tell her how broken-hearted she felt about her parents' broken marriage and how hard it was for her to put her feelings into words. Concurrently, the worker advised Lynnette's parents to stop trying to make her talk but rather to spend time with her, quietly acknowledging her expectable hurt and anger as appropriate.

At this point the worker met with the parents individually to assist them with their own sadness and anger about the ending of their relationship. She learned that the mother's father had died suddenly when Lynnette was 15 months old. This death left the mother profoundly depressed, in part because it occurred on her own birthday. Each year, the mother became despondent at the time of this powerful double anniversary. Lynnette, an only child who was sensitively tuned in to her mother's unresolved grief, annually saved up most of her allowance to buy her mother an expensive gift in hopes of "curing" her depression. Now, at the time of the mother's loss of another significant man in her life, Lynnette felt unable to ask for help with her own sadness, anger, and sense of abandonment. As the social worker took over the task of helping the mother with her grief, Lynnette gradually relinquished this role and began to turn to her mother for affection or for "someone to yell at when I feel mad." In a few months Lynnette's grades picked up, she seemed to be happier at school, and became more involved with friends. As the mother and father found a container for their own feelings in treatment, Lynnette no longer needed to "hold" them and could move on with her own individuation. She terminated with the understanding that she could return as needed.

INTERVENTION

Writing about the holding dimension of clinical social work, Saari (1991) notes that "when treatment is understood in this manner, it becomes clear that it will never be possible to reduce its principles to a set of techniques to be followed" (p. 169). Rather, each intervention will be uniquely and mutually constructed in the facilitating partnership between client and clinician. For Winnicott, such latitude was essential to creative clinical intervention and bespoke his allegiance to a constructivist approach to practice. Winnicott's three dimensions of the early caregiving activities—holding, handling, and object presenting—constitute a useful organizing framework for considering the holding environment as an aspect of intervention (Grolnick 1990).

Holding

As noted earlier, many types of concrete social services can be conceptualized in terms of their holding functions. The provision of food, clothing, housing, and financial assistance, for example, constitutes holding for many families seen in social agencies. Holding families together is a crucial aspect of child welfare services—an agenda that shapes the priorities of family preservation and other permanency planning programs. There are instances, however, when the holding function must be shifted outside the family. Under conditions of chronic abuse and neglect, for example, it may be possible to secure a "good-enough" holding environment only through removing children from their families of origin and arranging for alternative placement. Much of the work of foster care can be conceptualized in terms of finding and sustaining stable holding environments for children at risk.

Similarly, holding emerges as a central conceptual parameter of residential psychiatric treatment for children, adolescents, and adults. Gunderson (1978) specifies five holding dimensions of effective residential settings. The first is *containment*, related to the safety from external and internal impingements inherent in the rules, procedures, and boundaries of the hospital environment. Use of psychotropic medications to treat hallucinations can be viewed as a form of containment, as can the use of supervised seclusion for out-of-control patients in danger of harming themselves or others. *Support* ranges from provisions such as food, escorts, and entertainment, to specific direction, advice, education, and direct efforts to bolster reality testing and other ego functions. Support also finds expression in interventions such as praise and reassurance designed to enhance the client's self-esteem. *Structure* includes such parameters as daily schedules, chores, the hierarchy of statuses and privileges, and the reliability and predictability of relationships with staff members. *Involvement* promotes the holding dimension of the institutional community by encouraging clients to interact with fellow clients and staff members, and by examining intrapsychic phenomena in terms of their impact on the social milieu. For example, hallucinations, beyond being understood as intrapsychic phenomena, might be considered as an aspect of withdrawal from the community (Stamm 1985). Finally, *validation* interventions affirm each client's worth and individuality through encouraging activities that foster the development of unique talents and strengths.

In many other health and mental health settings there are certain points of transition where holding functions are central; yet they frequently become routinized and delegated to personnel who are not trained to be aware of their clinical significance. A medical hospital admission is a major disruption to the external holding environment and its internal representations. Hospital procedures and policies require patients to relinquish privacy and give themselves over to primary care by strangers. Such care inevitably promotes regression to dependence that stirs up early memories, feelings, and fantasies. Attention by admitting and nursing staff to these dynamics can ease patients' transition and provide opportunities for healing responses to their psychic as well as physical pain.

Similarly, discharge planning is a potentially traumatic transition that rarely receives the kind of attention it deserves. Often disparaged by social workers and hospital administrators as little more than glorified clerical work, discharge planning that takes into account the patient's psychodynamics requires sensitive, skillful assessment and intervention. It calls for assembling family and community holding structures and attending to the fears and uncertainties associated with leaving the carefully routinized life of the hospital. Planning for discharge, in other words, should be a process that makes room for reflection on its meaning to the patient and family so as to preserve the patient's internal sense of "going-on-being" as external circumstances change dramatically. Unfortunately, today's hospital policies, many driven by insurance imperatives, relate the timing of discharge more to fiscal timetables than to the patient's readiness to integrate the upheaval of departing the hospital. In some instances, patients are "dropped" from care precipitously, leading to anxieties in patients and families that can interfere with post-discharge recuperation. In these instances, social work follow-up is crucial.

Social workers in a host of other settings can conceptualize aspects of their roles and functions as creating and sustaining holding environments for clients. Those employed in employee assistance programs, for example, will see people whose work environment has been disrupted through layoffs or changes in assignments. Attention to the corollary disruptions in internal continuity helps focus intervention in a way that enables clients to reflect on the meaning of work-related changes. In family agencies, those working with couples who are separating or divorcing will also find the holding environment concept a useful clinical tool. Each partner's familiar relational context is being disrupted. Even when interactions have been primarily negative, relinquishing them is likely to be painful and evocative of separations from earlier objects. When children are involved, the clinician's awareness that their family holding environment is in flux can guide responsive intervention plans, as in Lynnette's case. This may include helping parents keep as much consistency as possible in the children's other important relationships and settings. Most parents have an intuitive understanding and recognition of the holding idea; formulating separation and divorce in these terms can help attune them to their children's needs and reactions.

Handling

Structural arrangements of the helping relationship are also part of the therapeutic holding environment. These are the containing boundaries of clinical work, and they find expression in the planned consistency of appointment times, the clear explication of policies and procedures related to planned absences or the cancellation of appointments, and, in most settings, arrangements related to fees. It is easy to underestimate the crucial significance of these parameters to the client's sense of the reliability and continuity of the helping relationship. It is especially difficult for beginning clinicians to understand that a client's wish to change or cancel an appointment may represent an unconscious effort to test the durability of the clinical holding environment. For clients whose lives have been characterized by inconsistency, too much flexibility can feel like a replication of earlier relationships that were insufficiently structured. In response, the client may act out his or her poorly integrated responses by failing to show for the newly scheduled appointment or in other ways "telling" the clinician through action what it feels like to have the framework of treatment altered. For example, a woman who had been unpredictably moved around from one foster home to another as a child reacted to her social worker's need to cancel an appointment by calling back and leaving a message that she was ending treatment.

This is not to say that clinicians should be rigid and ignore the changing realities of their own or their clients' lives; rather, the goal is to discuss and process any changes in terms of their many possible meanings to the client. Through such reflective conversation, clients can be helped to experience changes in the holding environment of treatment as aspects of an ongoing relational process rather than as unpredictable "events" over which they have little or no control.

Object Presenting

Winnicott spoke of object presenting as the way in which caregivers present the world of shared reality to the developing child. Similarly, the manner in which the clinician presents him- or herself and the treatment should convey the shared, collaborative nature of clinical work. This aspect of clinical holding finds expression in the clinician's demeanor and his or her use of self. Ideally, he or she should convey a calm, unhurried, receptive presence along with acceptance, a non-judgmental attitude, and respect for the

client's privacy. A social worker in a child guidance clinic
was reminded of the importance of this by a 5-year-old boy.
Having left herself too little time between sessions, she was
feeling pressured to end the boy's session on time. Sensing
her distractedness, the boy exclaimed angrily, "You're not a
worry doctor, you're a hurry doctor!"

Clinical holding requires time and willingness to listen,
an expressed desire to be helpful, and an effort to try to
understand the situation from the client's point of view. The
clinician's capacity to attend wholly to the client in this
manner is far more important than having quick answers
to the client's problem or being able to proffer clever interpretations. Such efforts to demonstrate expertise can interfere with the development of the mutual construction of the
clinical relationship—what Saari (1986) calls a therapeutic
"concordance" in which the client and the clinician "together
create and define the therapeutic culture within which they
work" (p. 210). To make concordance possible, the clinician
must, in Winnicott's sense, offer him- or herself as a potential subjective object for the client to discover or "find" rather
than as an omniscient expert who already knows all the
answers. The clinician needs to be willing to offer him- or
herself to be experienced in whatever way necessary to allow
for the past to be reconstructed in the present and thus made
available for *mutual* interpretation.

> Ms. E. came to the attention of the staff of a hospital pediat-
> ric unit when her first child, Tyrone, was admitted at age 15
> months with an arm fracture. When it was determined that she
> had inflicted this and other injuries on Tyrone, he was placed in
> temporary foster care pending a more thorough evaluation of
> Ms. E.'s ability to care for him. During the period of this evalu-
> ation, she became pregnant with a second child. Aware of the
> difficulties Ms. E. experienced in parenting Tyrone in his earli-
> est months, a team composed of doctors, nurses, and social
> workers in the pediatrics and obstetrics departments began an

intensive program of intervention designed to assist her in attaching to and nurturing her new baby. A protective services social worker and a lawyer from community legal services were also involved in this effort. For the duration of her pregnancy, Ms. E. was seen two to three times a week both in hospital offices and at home.

Ms. E. dutifully appeared for all her clinic and therapy appointments, reporting that, since Tyrone was no longer at home, she "had nothing better to do." Her compliance with this demanding schedule of appointments was striking. Gradually her story unfolded, narrated to the social worker in a fragmented, affectless manner that suggested a sense of resignation and little expectation that staff members would be interested in her. She was the youngest of four children, unplanned and unwanted, born to a mother who, as Ms. E. perceived it, was already emotionally depleted from taking care of the older children. Ms. E.'s mother seemed unable to protect either herself or the children from her husband's brutal beatings. Soon after Ms. E.'s birth, financial need required her mother to return to work, and she was left in the well-meaning but inconsistent care of various aunts and older siblings.

One of Ms. E.'s most striking characteristics was her sense of bewilderment. Sitting in the clinic waiting room or appearing at court hearings related to Tyrone's status, she seemed to have only a marginal grasp of what was going on around her. The social worker's assessment was that the unpredictable parade of caregivers of her infancy and early childhood had been unable to provide her with the reliable, consistent foundation of care she needed to begin to gather the bits and pieces of her early experience into a coherent pattern.

In initial sessions with the social worker, Ms. E. made very little eye contact. Her striking absence of response to the worker's efforts to make a connection gave the worker an eerie sense of not existing for her. The worker became doubtful about her ability to make a relationship with Ms. E., and she began to experience an urge to give up on her. The worker was surprised, therefore, that Ms. E. continued to keep her appointments. She remained puzzled by Ms. E.'s nonresponsiveness and her own sense of disconnection until, after two months of regular visits, Ms. E. gave her a clue: she began one appointment by asking, "When will I start seeing someone else?" In an instant the worker realized that Ms. E. expected their relationship to be short-lived; she had been compliantly waiting to be passed on to the next caregiver. For her there was no point in making a connection because it would soon be broken, repeating the fate of all the fragile bonds of her early life. The worker then understood that her urge to give up on Ms. E. and her sense of estrangement were expressions of countertransference. She had been experiencing empathically the depressive estrangement and lack of hope of continuity that characterized Ms. E.'s own object world. Ms. E.'s behavior was a form of communication that said, in effect, "By not engaging with you, I am giving you an experience of what I have experienced in other relationships."

After being reassured by the social worker that they would continue to work together, Ms. E. began to look at her face for the first time. As the worker approached her in the waiting room, Ms. E. would give a long, searching look accompanied by a deadpan facial expression; only when the worker smiled in greeting did Ms. E. risk a tentative smile of her own. This interaction constituted the first evidence that Ms. E. was beginning to engage in mirroring with the worker, thus taking one of the most basic first steps in establishing a relationship.

Ms. E. could not yet, however, consolidate enough of a sense of herself to take the initiative in mirroring interactions. It was this incapacity that continued to jeopardize her relationship with Tyrone. When visits were arranged, there would be a period when baby and mother sat looking warily at each other. As with the social worker, Ms. E. was unable to indicate that she was pleased to see Tyrone until he gave her some clue that he was pleased to see her. If no such clue appeared, she became angry and despondent, concluding that he did not care whether or not she came to see him. She would threaten to leave and not visit again. His seeming failure to acknowledge her existence made her doubt herself, filling her with rage and the impulse to strike out at him. Later it became clear that her rage acted as a defense: it protected her from the intolerable feeling that, without explicit positive responses from others, she did not exist.

At times she actively struggled with what Winnicott (1962a) referred to as the "unthinkable" anxiety associated with feelings of annihilation of the self. It was in such a state, triggered by Tyrone's unresponsiveness, that she had struck him with a broken chair leg and fractured his arm. Because her anxiety was "unthinkable," that is, unable to become an object of contemplation or reflection, it could be rendered more bearable only through impulsive action.

Not long after Ms. E. was reassured by the social worker that they could continue to work together through her pregnancy and beyond, Ms. E. began to come late for her appointments and then to miss one occasionally. The worker's sense was that Ms. E. was testing her durability as well as asking indirectly whether or not her presence mattered. On a couple of occasions she phoned during missed appointment times to find out if the worker were in her office or whether she had left to do something else. To the worker, this behavior signaled that Ms. E. had begun to be able to maintain a tentative image of the worker in her mind; and she needed to find out whether or not the worker held a corresponding image of her. Indeed, not only the worker but other members of the team were very much preoccupied with Ms. E. and her pregnancy. Great care was taken to assure that she saw the same doctor and nurse on each of her visits. Everyone involved worked to create a continuity and stability designed to affirm for Ms. E. that she did exist and had meaning for others. The primary agenda was to avoid a repetition of the environmental failure she had sustained as an infant.

As part of an effort to "hold" the entire family, the team reached out actively to the baby's father. He attended childbirth preparation classes with Ms. E. and took pride in his abilities as a delivery coach. Having seen a movie in which a cab driver had to deliver a baby in a taxi, he began to do some reading on his own in case the baby arrived before he could get Ms. E. to the hospital. With both parents the team did as much as possible to promote attachment to the expected child. Both took delight in an ultrasound and, because the father liked to sing, he was encouraged to sing lullabies when the baby was moving and kicking in utero. At first, Ms. E. complained about the kicking, experiencing it as an act of aggression against her. The team reframed this for her in terms of the baby's beginning exploration of the world and efforts to begin to connect with Ms. E.

When baby Susan did arrive the team waited in trepidation to see what she would bring of her own—would she be active, quiet, fussy, connect easily? To everyone's relief she was alert and engaging, observing the world around her with large dark eyes. In the five days before Ms. E. and Susan left the hospital, there were intensive interventions designed to promote their attachment. This effort involved the resident who delivered Susan, the nursing staff both in obstetrics and in the high risk nursery, and the social work staff. They noted that, while Ms. E. was quite adept at handling the baby, she did so in an efficient but distant and perfunctory way. The staff modeled primary maternal preoccupation for Ms. E., coaxing her into joining them in studying Susan's face and marveling over the perfection of her fingers and toes. They affirmed what a fine job she had done in producing such a beautiful infant.

Since Ms. E. lived in housing projects near the hospital it was easy for the social worker to visit her twice a week until she was able to resume office visits. The resident working in the high risk nursery developed a close relationship to her and gave her his home phone number with encouragement to call as needed. Ms. E. did better than predicted in her mothering of Susan, in all likelihood due to the staff's combined efforts to provide her with a holding environment she could count on. Things did not go as well with Tyrone; the early disruptions in Ms. E.'s relationship to him and insufficient intervention while he was in foster care left him at continued risk.

When Susan was 8 months old, the family moved to another part of the city and the hospital team lost touch with them. The team felt successful, however, in having provided a facilitating partnership with Ms. E. that enabled her to hold Susan securely during her crucial first eight months. The staff noted that they had forged strong bonds with each other as well; there were frequent meetings and telephone contacts. In essence they had constructed a supportive holding environment for themselves that sustained their hope and mission through the ups and downs of this intensive intervention.

As Grolnick (1990) succinctly puts it, and as illustrated by this and other cases in this chapter, "holding comes first" (p. 144). It constitutes the therapeutic matrix for all other clinical activity. In Ms. E.'s case, the holding was multidisciplinary and required much intra- and interprofessional collaboration. It called on representatives of the child welfare and legal systems as well as a number of health professionals. The complex orchestration of services, clinical and otherwise, is a frequent task of social workers in many settings. Here, holding moves from the dyadic level of clinical social work to the family system to larger community systems. Ultimately, we can conceptualize agency policies and procedures and, in a broader sense, social policy formation and implementation in terms of the extent to which they hold the people they are intended to serve. If holding is adequate and affirming, ego relatedness follows.

5

EGO RELATEDNESS

When the social worker has successfully "held" the beginning helping relationship "so that growth tendencies are given a chance" (Winnicott 1961, p. 107), the stage is set for the emergence of clinical ego relatedness. Winnicott (1956a) noted that, out of the matrix of a good-enough caregiving environment, "There comes into existence an ego relatedness between mother and baby" that permits the baby to "build the idea of a person in the mother" (p. 304). Similarly, if the social worker has been able to sustain the treatment relationship beyond the initial contact or contacts, an opportunity for the client to construct a personal idea of the worker, and vice versa, is at hand.

When Winnicott (1960d) declared that "there is no such thing as an infant" (p. 39), he spoke about the *person* of the infant. He meant that only in a facilitating partnership with a caregiver could the baby come into existence as a social being. Although he did not do so, Winnicott might also have added, "there is no such thing as a mother," thus giving voice to the reality that, without a baby, the mother qua mother would not exist. Transposing this idea of fundamental dialectical mutuality to clinical work, we can say there is no such thing as a client, and, without a client, no such thing as a clinician. This concept does not negate the existence of two individuals in distinct roles; but the focus falls on the relationship as the primary motivational context for clinical practice. The facilitating partnership emerges as central. In the context of this partnership, each participant builds an idea of the other that is shaped in part by experiences with previous significant objects. Hence, Winnicott (1958) refers to ego relatedness as the matrix of transference, and, we would add, the matrix of countertransference. But in addition, client and clinician build new and unique conceptions of each other on the basis of their present-day "real" relationship—out of the intersubjective knowledge that unfolds in the process of getting to know each other. The developmental dialectic between merger and autonomy finds expression as each party notes, and registers internally, their similarities and differences.

A 3-year-old African-American child entered a white social worker's office for their first appointment. As the worker bent down to introduce herself, the boy reached up and touched her face. After about a minute of silent visual and tactile exploration, he said, "You are pink. I am brown. You have boo-boo on your face. I have boo-boo on my thumb. My hair is black. Your hair is not black. What is your name?"

Another client, Mr. M., found it awkward to look at his social worker but was keenly aware of the sound and rhythm of her voice. He grew up in the hills of Kentucky and spoke with a thick southern drawl, while she spoke with a pronounced British accent. After the worker spent several minutes outlining services the agency could offer Mr. M. and his family, she was surprised that he made no reply. Instead he sat quietly, a rapt expression on his face. When the worker asked what Mr. M. thought about what she had just said, he looked startled and confessed he had not understood a word, "but your voice sure sounded pretty—just like my mamma's when it got dark and she'd start croonin' to the baby."

As noted in Chapter 2, Winnicott (1958) employed paradox to express the dialectical nature of ego relatedness: "Ego-relatedness refers to the relationship between two people, one of whom at any rate is alone; perhaps both are alone, yet the presence of each is important to the other" (p. 31). Only when alone *in the presence of someone*, he believed, could the infant discover his or her unique personal life. This capacity to sustain a solid sense of oneself as a distinct person while in the intimate presence of another depends on early experiences with caregivers who are attentive, supportive, and non-intrusive, permitting interpersonal space for the child's "going-on-being" and welcoming his or her spontaneous gestures. Winnicott believed that, over time, the child internalizes soothing aspects of ego relatedness and gradually becomes able to experience internal continuity and safety without someone else present. This structuralization is the result of the transitional process, whose clinical implications will be considered in the next chapter.

Winnicott (1958) coined the term *ego relatedness* to capture what he observed in very young infants—observations that have since been validated repeatedly in the burgeoning body of research on infancy of the past twenty years. In contrast to Freud's assertion that the first few weeks and months of life are characterized by id-relatedness or primary narcissism, protected from outside influence by a stimulus barrier, Winnicott (1962a) saw evidence of ego functioning from the beginning: "Is there an ego from the start? The answer is that the start is when the ego starts" (p. 56). Kestenberg (1978) has since coined the term *transsensus* to

describe what Winnicott saw: a "going out of one's boundaries and incorporating others" (p. 66), a stretching outward
so that the body "becomes imbued with a feeling of vitality,
as if life were flowing through it" (p. 65).

This stretching toward others calls for a response, or
relatedness—a behavioral acknowledgement that something
important is being taken in and registered by the other party
in the interaction. There are efforts to share attention, intention, and feelings preverbally as well as an expectation
of—indeed a demand for—reciprocation. In the absence of
a response, the psyche regresses to id phenomena which, in
the absence of ego relatedness, become disintegrative and
disruptive of internal continuity. In a film entitled *Life's
First Feelings* (Lipscomb and Wander 1986), the viewer sees
an infant and his mother in playful interaction. In response
to her baby's alert readiness to interact, the mother moves
in to vocalize in an animated way and tickle him around the
chin and face. After a time, this stimulation appears to be
too much for the infant and, apparently temporarily satu-
rated, he turns his head to the side and appears to disen-
gage, to take a break. Soon, he looks back to the mother's
face, and smiles to signal his readiness for more stimulating play. Having waited patiently for her baby's readiness
to resume interaction, the mother now moves in again to
tickle, vocalize, and in other ways mirror and affirm his delight and his capacity to engage her. Mother and baby are
partners in a mutually attuned affective and behavioral
dance, choreographed according to oscillating periods of
intense engagement and periods of "time out."

To demonstrate the effects on the infant of stretching toward relatedness and not finding an attuned response, the
researcher asks the mother to remain silent and to present
an expressionless face to the baby when, after a time out,
he looks to her for a resumption of their lively interaction.
The effects of the mother's frozen countenance on the baby's

behavior are striking and immediate. At first, the excited grin falters. Seeing that the mother is not responding to him, he turns away, looks back hopefully, then, appearing perplexed, looks away again. Soon he begins to drool, seeming to lose control of functions that have been easily regulated to this point. He becomes fidgety and physically uncomfortable, arching his body and appearing to withdraw in an autistic manner. Finally, seeming to register fully that the mother is not going to respond, disintegration appears total; his face contorts painfully and he begins to sob uncontrollably. The researcher likens the baby's profoundly sad expression to that of the babies in Spitz's studies of institutionalized infants, some of whom eventually died as a result of isolation and emotional deprivation.

Viewers find reassurance in the knowledge that this sequence is only an experiment; soon the mother will respond, and this baby will return to his previous interactive exhilaration. But the effects of a chronic absence or disturbance of ego relatedness are profound and long-lasting, often leading people to drastic behaviors in their efforts to exact some response from the human environment. Some researchers (Applegate and Barol 1989, McGee et al. 1987) suggest that this concept helps explain the severe behavior disorders observed in people with developmental disabilities and mental retardation. Such behaviors as hitting, spitting, random screaming, head banging, rocking, fecal smearing, and hair pulling appear to be related primarily to impaired mental capacity or other neurological phenomena. This understanding frequently leads to interventions based on social learning strategies designed to produce rapid behavior modification. Although behavior change is a primary goal with these distressed and distressing clients, an exclusive focus on behavior change constricts the parameters of intervention and reduces opportunities for psychological change and personal growth.

Rather than viewing autistic, combative, and self-abusive behaviors as secondary to retardation per se, developmentally oriented clinician-researchers view them as secondary to major disruptions in bonding and ego relatedness. While incorporating techniques intended to reinforce positive behaviors, their overall approach is grounded in primary attention to the clinician-client relationship. This approach reframes the clinical task from behavior management to "gentle teaching" based on the rewards inherent in human presence and participation (McGee et al. 1987). By attending to derivatives of disruptions in earliest ego relatedness, clinical interventions can lay the groundwork for enhanced adaptation and further social and emotional development. While benefitting clients, this focus also helps clinicians feel more engaged and empathic in ways that reduce discouragement and burnout.

This approach requires an understanding of what can happen to ego relatedness when the baby's developmental vulnerabilities interfere with its accomplishment. In retardation and related difficulties, the impairment in constitutional cognitive and sensory capacities causes a slowing down in responses. Both in responding to caregivers' overtures and in initiating interactions with them, infants with retardation are frustratingly slow, often appearing bland, tuned-out, and disconnected. This slowed and blunted responsiveness disrupts the "dance" of parent–infant mutuality so crucial to psychosocial development. Moreover, when parents' worst fears come true in the form of a damaged neonate, enormous guilt can be mobilized. This guilt can lead to depression and emotional withdrawal from the baby. Even basic interactions such as feeding can become disengaged and mechanistic. Caregivers of these infants may feed them without looking at their faces, thus reducing opportunities for the mirroring interactions that form the template for later expressive communication. Deprived of the chance to see the caregiver's facial animation and learn its nuances, many of these babies evince disturbances in affective expression and regulation that range from emotional blandness to hyperkinetic agitation. Left psychologically alone, without the internalized structure to provide self-soothing, some of these babies appear to be flooded with the "unbearable agonies" Winnicott referred to so frequently. Their tuned-out or frantic behaviors have the effect of pushing caregivers away further. Caregiver withdrawal generates more anxiety in the baby, and the cycle of misattunement and failed ego relatedness begins anew.

ASSESSMENT AND INTERVENTION BASED ON EGO RELATEDNESS

As older children and adults, people whose early years have been characterized by severely impaired ego relatedness present special challenges to those attempting clinical work with them. In many instances effective assessment and intervention turn on the way in which clinicians can use the therapeutic relationship to establish and sustain ego relatedness, often a new and frightening experience for clients. The clinician learns to attend to his or her own inner life as a source of clues about how to approach troubled clients. Operating interpersonally on the basis of an inadequately integrated sense of self and others, these clients may behave in ways that replicate earlier experiences of being psychologically "dropped." They frequently present themselves in a manner that repulses and drives away others, ignoring personal hygiene and appearing dirty and disheveled. They may hit, kick, spit, or self-mutilate as ways of both provoking external control from and experiencing some sense of engagement with others. Their compromised capacity for self-regulation can also find expression in attempts to share positive emotions; they may hug too hard or laugh too loudly. Overwhelmed by these behaviors, clinicians may find it difficult to sustain a developmental understanding of them. Countertransference issues abound. Clinicians, like the parents, may be put in touch with their own long-denied and repressed primitive fears and instinctual impulses. In an effort to manage the uncomfortable feelings generated by these impulses, they may retreat from the relationship in ways that disrupt the empathic matrix.

Difficulties with Primary Attachment

Mrs. S., a 45-year-old state hospital patient, attended daily group therapy sessions as part of her treatment for chronic schizophrenia. For the first week after her admission, every time another patient or a staff member mentioned feelings of sadness or loss, Mrs. S. would rock vigorously while laughing wildly. At such times the group leader, an experienced social worker who felt overwhelmed both by this bizarre behavior and the distress it caused the group, would ask another staff member to escort Mrs. S. from the room. Mrs. S. would exit only with force, all the while screaming profanities. After consultation with a senior colleague, the worker began to sit next to Mrs. S. during group meetings. When she began rocking, he would do the same, telling the group that Mrs. S. was showing them with her whole body how much it pained her to hear about sad feelings. Instead of laughing, Mrs. S. began to cry. Again, she was loud and wailed in a grotesque way that frightened others in the group. Several entreated the social worker to remove her from the group. The worker persisted, talking about the depth of Mrs. S.'s pain and empathizing with the group about their degree of disturbance at such open displays of intense feeling. After several sessions Mrs. S. began to share her distress by moaning. Group members could tolerate and respond sympathetically to this behavior. Mrs. S. then was able to use this new way of showing her painful feelings to her family, enabling them to respond empathically rather than retreat in anger as they had done in the past.

One manifestation of this retreat in clinicians is a fragmented ego relatedness that focuses intervention on changing specific behavioral fragments presented by the client. This focus seems to justify the use of distancing—even aversive—behavior modification techniques. Resulting clinical postures can range from infantilizing overprotectiveness to authoritarian tactics. Reframing clients' disordered behaviors as misdirected attempts at self-soothing and ego relatedness can set the stage for gentle teaching of behaviors more likely to foster mutuality and its attendant developmental rewards.

> Ms. M., a tall, overweight, unkempt 27-year-old woman with a dual diagnosis of mental retardation and psychosis, lived in a community residence with six other developmentally challenged adults. She had lived in institutions since early childhood. Despite staff members' attempts at behavior management and the prescription of various combinations of psychotropic medications, Ms. M. frequently tyrannized staff and other residents with unpredictable episodes of destructive behavior. In addition to hitting, spitting on, and screaming at others, she hit herself, ripped her clothes, forced herself to vomit, and had toilet accidents. Repulsed, angered, and fearful, staff members resorted to increasingly restrictive aversive behavior modification techniques, including seclusion and restraint, that appeared to intensify rather than reduce Ms. M.'s distress.
>
> Feeling depleted and helpless, the staff came as a group to implore the residence administrator, a clinical social worker, to remove Ms. M. and place her in a more restrictive setting. Once given the opportunity to talk about the depth of their revulsion and their sense of being contenders in a tug-of-war they could never win, staff members could begin to consider the social worker's suggestion that Ms. M.'s behavior might be a cry for connectedness rather than an invitation to combat. After much discussion, they agreed to an approach whose objective was to promote non-adversarial bonding between Ms. M. and her caregivers.

The social worker began an intensive ten-day period of direct work with Ms. M. and educative consultation with staff members. For staff she conceptualized Ms. M.'s behavior in psychodynamic developmental terms that emphasized the vicissitudes of disrupted infant–caregiver mutuality. They were helped to view Ms. M.'s infantile behaviors as negatively reinforced attempts to engage them in close interaction and as misdirected efforts at self-stimulation. Screaming, self-abuse, and clothes-ripping were conceptualized as manifestations of primitive unbearable anxiety related to feeling psychologically "dropped" and abandoned. Her poor hygiene was viewed both as a sign of low self-esteem and of being out of touch with her body. Her enraged contentiousness was reframed as a plea for interrelatedness.

As they understood this reformulation, staff members felt increased empathy for Ms. M. and were less self-critical. They saw themselves less as failed helpers and more as partners in an affectively dyssynchronous relationship orchestrated by Ms. M.'s misdirected attempts to engage the world around her. This revised perspective was crucial preparation for learning a new approach—one that began with lifting all of Ms. M.'s restraints and eliminating her periods of seclusion.

A priority for beginning to work with Ms. M. was paying attention to her hygiene and grooming. The obvious advantage was to make her more approachable by staff who had been repulsed by her odor and unkempt appearance. As the social worker viewed it, however, attention to hygiene was also an avenue for helping Ms. M. get in touch with her body in positive, soothing ways. Staff members were supported in helping her bathe. The importance of gentle touch and quiet conversation was emphasized as part of the bathing experience. Hairbrushing was seen as an opportunity to help Ms. M. feel comfortable with rhythmic stroking by another. Gradually, Ms. M. was encouraged to groom herself while someone else was present. She appeared to take delight at her new image in the mirror and in the positive responses from those around her.

Drawing on an understanding of the feeding experience as a pivotal developmental interaction, the social worker then helped members change their interventions related to Ms. M.'s primitive oral cravings and behaviors. Staff were particularly upset by Ms. M.'s insatiable demands for tea, coffee, and soft drinks. At the residence and during trips into the community, she snatched soft drinks from others, screamed loudly, and often assaulted them. Prior to the social worker's intervention, staff members' response was to punish Ms. M. by depriving her of all her favorite beverages. In frantic reaction, she then scrounged in garbage pails for and ate coffee grounds and tea bags.

Helped to view these behaviors as derivatives of a thirst for emotional nurturance, staff members shifted from a posture of behavior control to one intended to produce interpersonal reward. As their empathy increased, they became more aware of things they liked about Ms. M. They paid attention less to the number of times she spit and screamed and more to the number of times she smiled, reached out, or tried a new task. Regardless of her behavior during the day, Ms. M. received the reward of a soft drink every evening after her shower. At first amazed at this consistency, she gradually learned to trust that the soft drink would be proffered unconditionally. Her inappropriate cravings for beverages decreased in tandem with the increase in her level of trust.

A conscious use of the dynamics of the feeding situation also guided the social worker's direct interventions with Ms. M. They met in daily sessions lasting up to three hours. At their first meeting, they sat down to a snack together. Toward the end of this session, Ms. M. was invited to place a cracker on the worker's lips, causing her to look into the worker's face and make eye contact. In subsequent meetings, the worker helped Ms. M. learn how to prepare meals. Bonding, rather than task completion, was the primary focus of each activity. Throughout the painstaking work of teaching Ms. M. how to make a salad, the social worker provided verbal and gestural praise as often as forty times a minute: "Good! That's great, tearing the lettuce; fantastic, chopping the cucumber; that's right, pour in some more dressing!" This enthusiastic support was punctuated by hugs, kisses, stroking, and other physical praise and reinforcement.

Of course, at times Ms. M. became acutely anxious during these sessions and regressed to disruptive behavior. The worker's tactic when Ms. M. began to scream, hit, or rip her

clothes was to re-direct her back to the task at hand and reward her for returning to the task and to the interaction, moving in and out of range as necessary. Occasionally, Ms. M.
wandered away from activities to rock gently on her feet from
side to side, appearing to enter a trance. Rather than interrupt
this obvious attempt at rhythmic self-soothing, the social
worker stood in front of Ms. M., rocking with her and gazing
into her face to make eye contact. Gradually, Ms. M. sustained
longer periods of eye contact and began to mirror the worker's
facial expressions.

At other times Ms. M.'s enthusiasm at successfully complet-
ing a task spilled over and caused her to hug the worker too
tightly and aggressively while jumping up and down. Previously
such behavior had prompted staff members to place Ms. M. on
a "no hugging" program. In contrast, the social worker first
praised Ms. M. and thanked her for the hug; then she suggested,
"Now try hugging me this way," while positioning Ms. M.'s arms
appropriately and calming her. Then, "Oh, this is a good hug; I
love getting this kind of hug from you." Subsequently, Ms. M.
frequently returned to the worker for the ego relatedness of good
hugging.

At first there appeared to be little carry-over of these behavior
gains between sessions with the social woker. It was necessary
for the worker to intrude into Ms. M.'s autistic-appearing
behaviors at the beginning of each session to reestablish ego
relatedness. Gradually, however, an internalized sense of safety
enabled her to "remember" the worker and relate more immediately. The successful repetition of meal preparations and other
self-care tasks helped Ms. M. feel more in control of her daily
life. This external control appeared to facilitate internal control over the intensity of her anxiety.

The initial ten-day period of the social worker's direct intervention both offered Ms. M. an experience in ego relatedness and
modeled this approach for other residence staff members. Gradually, the social worker reduced the frequency of her contacts with
Ms. M. in order to foster primary attachment to residence staff.
The capacity for ego relatedness transferred smoothly to others,
and the social worker's role shifted to one of support through
weekly consultation. Within two months, Ms. M.'s disruptive be-

haviors decreased dramatically, diminished not through external control but through internalized positive relatedness.

As the staff took more pleasure in Ms. M.'s accomplishments, they talked about them in much the same way that a mother crows about the triumphs of her practicing toddler. Building on the interpersonal skills developed with staff members, Ms. M. made more friends among other residents. Today, on a small maintenance dosage of medication, Ms. M. enjoys coffee, tea, and soft drinks while sitting down with her friends at the residence. The frequency of staff meetings about Ms. M. has diminished to one "pep rally" per month.

In Ms. M.'s case, what at first appeared to be pure id relatedness was reframed by the social worker as a repertoire of misdirected attempts at ego relatedness. Using Winnicott's ideas, she viewed Ms. M.'s maladaptive behaviors as spontaneous gestures —strangely expressed but very human efforts to try herself out in the world. When these gestures were unmet or rejected, she turned to behaviors that ranged from self-stimulation and autistic reverie to intrusive, attention-demanding attacks on others. Apparently having been left alone in institutions before being able to construct reliable mental representations of soothing others, Ms. M. found ways to assure that others would relate to her, even if aversively. To begin to redirect her attempts at relatedness into more mutually gratifying interactions, the social worker employed methods based on an understanding of the organizing qualities of earliest infant–caregiver interactions. Activities such as bathing and hair brushing served as opportunities for residence staff members to help Ms. M. experience positive body-skin sensations in a comfortable interpersonal context. Even after years of stimulating herself in primarily painful ways, Ms. M. appeared to learn the value of gentle, soothing touch very quickly. Similarly, the social worker used the social ritual of sharing food as a means of establishing ego relatedness with Ms. M. By asking Ms. M. to "feed" her with a cracker, the worker drew on her knowl-

edge of the infant's first spontaneous gestures to affirm Ms.
M.'s worth as someone who had something valuable to give
to others. The worker extended the benefits of this fundamental contact by helping Ms. M. learn how to prepare and
serve food, thus offering the secondary benefit of promoting her autonomy and self-sufficiency.

Just as parents are able to respond adaptively to a responsive, engaging infant, Ms. M.'s caregivers and fellow residents responded positively to her increased sense of self and
her growing vitality. They reported less discouragement and,
rather than adversaries, they became Ms. M.'s cheerleaders.
In part, this transformation resulted from the social worker's
acceptance of staff members' original negative feelings toward Ms. M. as legitimate and understandable. Just as parents of impaired children cannot be blamed for withdraw-
ing from them, caregivers of clients with behavior disorders
cannot be blamed for their negative responses. When they
come to understand that their revulsion or withdrawal is
evidence of a fundamental misattunement in which the
client plays a part, caregivers experience less guilt and become more empathic. Furthermore, the establishment of
ego relatedness as the primary focus of intervention while
making task accomplishment secondary reduces burnout by
allowing staff members to relate more flexibly and positively
to clients. This approach is humanizing and liberating for
clients and caregivers alike.

The Involuntary Client

Establishing ego relatedness with involuntary clients can
also present a formidable challenge. When people seek help
voluntarily, even though there may be resistance initially and
at various points in the helping process, they generally bring
at least a willingness to engage with the clinician. When such
willingness is absent but legal requirements mandate intervention, the clinician must be particularly adept and creative
in finding ways to invite the client into a productive rela-

tionship. It can be argued, of course, that even involuntary clients, through behaving in ways that call them to the attention of legal or other regulatory systems, unconsciously set up conditions that ensure professional intervention. In such situations we might say that clients' drive for ego relatedness finds expression in acting-out. They use the language of action, in other words, to signal that they need assistance. Characteristically, however, conscious awareness of such motivation is absent, and involuntary clients often bring mistrust, fear, and hostility to their initial contacts with helping professionals.

Ms. C., a 29-year-old African-American single mother, was referred for social work consultation by a pediatrician who saw her in an inner-city hospital emergency room. She had brought her 2-year-old son, Tommy, for treatment of a severe burn on his arm, alleged by her to have resulted from his "messing around" with a pot of boiling water on the stove. The pediatrician noted, however, that the burn followed a glove-like pattern, suggesting that Tommy's arm had been intentionally held in scalding water. In such instances hospital policy required admitting the child as a protective measure while the suspicion of abuse was investigated by the hospital's protective services team. It fell to the social worker to inform the family of these policies and procedures and to report the suspected abuse to the child protective unit of the department of public welfare. From the outset, then, the social worker faced the challenge of establishing an alliance with a person whom she was required to "turn in" to an agency viewed by members of the community as punitive and focused on removing children from their families.

Prior to meeting with Ms. C., the social worker's brief consultation with the emergency room nurse and the referring pediatrician revealed that Ms. C. was sullen, uncooperative, and hostile. Her apparent nonchalance about Tommy's injury had aroused feelings of outrage in the staff. The social worker quickly became aware of images of Ms. C. as angry and unfeeling. She felt reluctant to meet Ms. C., expecting that her overtures would be rebuffed. She took a few moments to let these images and feelings develop in her mind. As she did so, she began to consider that her own feelings might be mirroring those of Ms. C. as she sat waiting to meet this stranger who might arrange to have her son taken away. Perhaps Ms. C. had begun to imagine the social worker to be punitive and unfeeling as well. Equipped with increased empathy for Ms. C.'s possible feelings, the social worker entered the emergency room cubicle to introduce herself.

Her first glimpse of mother and child suggested a probable disturbance in their relationship. Tommy lay listlessly on the bed, his head turned toward Ms. C., who sat on a chair in the corner furthest from him, filing her nails. This tableau evoked strong maternal feelings in the social worker, who fought impulses to comfort the boy or urge his mother to do so. Instead, she noted the detachment as a portent that forming a connection with Ms. C. might be a formidable task.

Hypothesizing that her distance from Tommy might be an expression of Ms. C.'s discomfort with physical closeness, the social worker took a chair at as much distance from her as the confining space of the small cubicle would allow. In an effort to acknowledge and support Ms. C.'s strengths as a mother, the worker began: "I'm glad that you brought Tommy in so quickly. You were right to realize that the burn on his arm is severe and needs medical attention." Ms. C. remained silent, but the worker detected a flicker of surprise in her eyes and a slight softening of her stony facial expression as she slowly put her nail file away.

In a second overture intended to speak to Ms. C.'s strengths, the social worker said that, in glancing at the medical chart, she had noticed that the family lived a great distance from the hospital and that bringing Tommy by bus must have been difficult for her to do alone. Ms. C. snapped back angrily that she was used to doing things alone: "I'd have called the cops to bring me, but they ask too many questions." The social worker noted the communication to her that was implicit in this statement: the people who are supposed to help cannot be trusted. Ms. C. continued, "All I want is to get out of here—I'm tired of waiting around for all these people to poke their noses in my business. I brought my kid here to have his arm fixed and now that that's done I want to go home and get some rest." She then stood up and picked up her coat. The social worker felt challenged and had a sense of the importance of standing her ground.

Ms. C.'s belligerence appeared to be her way of taking charge of a situation that made her feel vulnerable, frightened, and out of control. Her response to the anxiety aroused by these feelings was to strike out at the worker and then flee. To help Ms. C. contain rather than act out this anxiety and to preserve contact with the part of her that had reached out by bringing Tommy to the hospital, the social worker concentrated on providing a firm, calm presence. Remaining seated, she said that Ms. C. did look tired and that she had been through a lot: "Nevertheless, we do need to talk further about Tommy. Then you will be able to go home." The social worker noticed heavy nicotine stains on Ms. C.'s fingers and surmised that smoking might be one way she soothed herself. Since smoking was not permitted in the emergency room, she invited Ms. C. to her office where she could smoke and have more privacy. With a cigarette and a snack, Ms. C. appeared to calm down.

As she ate, Ms. C. did sustain eye contact with the social worker. This took the form of a hostile glare, but the worker's sense was that a beginning connection was being forged. The disdainful stare hardened as the social worker explained that Tommy would be admitted to the hospital and that, because the emergency room staff suspected that Tommy's burn did not happen accidentally, she was required to file a report of suspected child abuse to the child welfare department. The social worker paused to give Ms. C. an opportunity to respond. She remained stonily silent, maintaining her angry visage. The worker continued, describing services that the hospital offered families. She commented that, while it might not seem that she and the other staff could be of help, other families in similar situations had been helped: "Letting yourself trust me even a little may feel very frightening right now. Perhaps it seems like others have let you down, but it needn't always be that way." Ms. C. responded with a derisive "Huh!" To the social worker it seemed positive that Ms. C. had listened and responded to her at all. She proceeded: "It must be hard for you to imagine anything good coming of all this. I have a sense, though, that there has been a lot of upset in your life even before Tommy's arm got burned. I wonder if you even hoped that someone would understand that and give you a chance to get some help with it. Perhaps while Tommy's in the hospital you could begin to tell me some of what you've been going through."

For the next few days Ms. C. came to visit Tommy in the early evening. The nursing staff reported that she rejected overtures from them, but they did observe her talking and playing with Tommy, who seemed quite responsive to her. The social worker telephoned Ms. C. daily, expressing her concern and commenting on her flat, tired voice. To questions about her depression, Ms. C. responded that she was sleeping a great deal during the day and that she had been hospitalized for depression several years ago. At the social worker's urging, she reluctantly accepted an appointment with one of the hospital psychiatrists. The social worker recognized Ms. C.'s request that she accompany her to the appointment as a significant step in the development of their relationship.

Prior to this appointment, Ms. C. came in for a second session with the social worker. She appeared more depressed; her hair was straggly and uncombed, and she wore no makeup. Her gait was markedly slowed, the glare was gone, and her eyes were downcast except for a momentary glance when the social worker greeted her. She appeared to be in an inaccessible other world. The social worker reached out by using Ms. C.'s first name: "Rhonda, do you remember me?" Ms. C. looked up slowly and nodded. When the worker commented about how sad she looked, tears began to trickle down Ms. C.'s face. When asked if she could put some of her feelings into words, she shook her head. Indeed, her desolation appeared to be beyond words. Noticing the body language of Ms. C.'s posture and slowed movement, the social worker said, "You look as though you feel so weighed down by your sadness that it is hard for you to move, let alone talk. Perhaps you feel there is no hope of things getting any better, that nothing you do or say will make a difference, so why try?" Ms. C. nodded again. "It may seem like the safest thing to do is to keep everything to yourself so you can't ever be hurt again. If this is how you are feeling, I am sure there are good reasons and, maybe if you can get to know me better, you'll be able to tell me what they are." Ms. C. shook her head in resignation, as though this could never be. She did, however, reestablish eye contact, this time a bit longer than previously. The social worker continued, "Rhonda, I wonder if maybe you would really like to believe there is some hope but are afraid to try and risk being disappointed again." As Ms. C. nodded in agreement, fresh tears streamed down her face.

Accompanied by Tommy's father and the social worker, Ms. C. came in for psychiatric consultation. She was very frightened, saying that the last time she had seen a psychiatrist, following the removal from home of her other four children, she was hospitalized with "a lot of crazy people" and felt worse. She believed that the hospitalization had been used against her in court when she tried to get her children back. The social worker responded, "I know this sometimes happens and when it does it feels like a terrible betrayal, like you are being punished for trying to do the right thing. I would not let that happen again. When the court hearing comes up to decide what will happen when Tommy leaves the hospital, I will be there, along with your attorney. Your willingness to get psychiatric help before was very positive. I don't think you can take care of Tommy in the way you would like to while you're feeling so depressed, but I do feel confident that the depression can be treated. Medication is a possibility. Perhaps the doctor will suggest hospitalization, but you can choose to try outpatient treatment first. In any case, it may be that you won't be able to take Tommy home right away, but I do think we can help you so that you are able to take care of him again." As it turned out, the psychiatrist felt Ms. C. could be treated as an outpatient and prescribed antidepressant medication.

A full pediatric, neurological, and psychological evaluation revealed that Tommy was a well-nourished youngster with only slight developmental delays in the area of expressive language. He had been able to make a good attachment to his primary nurse and, while he was exhibiting signs of depression, they appeared to be reactions to the recent abuse rather than to a chronic process. Absence of profound disturbance gave reason to hope that Tommy was constitutionally sturdy and had experienced some adequate holding during his first two years. On the basis of these strengths in the situation, the evaluation team recommended work toward his return home rather than long-term foster placement.

To lay the groundwork for this plan and to demonstrate a willingness to reach out to Ms. C., the hospital's child protective services team arranged four sessions of in-home treatment with the social worker. When the worker arrived for the first appointment, Ms. C. opened the door so quickly that it seemed she had been standing right by it, waiting. She did not respond verbally to the worker's greeting but motioned her to sit on a couch in the living room and then positioned herself at the other end. After brief discussion of some side effects of Ms. C.'s medication, the social worker asked, "How did you feel about my coming here today?" Ms. C. sighed, then fell silent. When the worker commented on the sigh, Ms. C. only shrugged. Attending to her own discomfort with the silence, the worker waited a while before beginning to try to give words to what she imagined Ms. C. might be feeling. "I don't know if this is right, but I have the sense that you feel like giving up, that Tommy has been taken from you, like your other children were, and you are convinced that you can never get him back. Could it be that you are afraid to hope that things will get better, and that not hoping is a way to protect yourself from being let down again?" Ms. C. then looked at the worker and nodded. The worker continued, "I can't promise you anything, but I can tell you that it does not have to be that way. We have been able to help other families get back together again. I know that it is hard for you to take the risk of letting someone help you, and fighting your depression is going to be tough, but you don't have to do it alone this time."

Ms. C. turned to stare out the window, replying, "Well, there ain't going to be anybody here. Tommy's dad says I'm too evil to be around, always going off at him for nothing. My mom hangs up when I call and she's turned the kids against me. That woman from the child welfare says she can't help if I won't talk to her. Ain't going to be no different this time." Choosing her words carefully, the social worker replied, "I guess you think that I am going to give up on you too. True, if you don't let yourself get involved you can't get hurt more, but you are left all alone with the hurt you're already feeling. I can't help but feel, though, that you do have a little hope. It's true that you don't talk much, but you do talk a little. I don't think your not talking means that you can't or don't want to be helped. Perhaps we just have to be patient until talking feels safer to you." Ms. C. sighed again, lapsing into silence. After a while, the worker continued: "It must feel like a no-win situation. If you tell me how you really feel, including how angry you are, I'll leave, and if you keep these feelings to yourself I'll quit on you because you won't talk." Seeming to mull this idea over, Ms. C. eventually mumbled, "Talking just gets you into trouble." When the social worker wondered how so, Ms. C. shook her head. She barely spoke for the remainder of their time together, but somehow the silence felt more comfortable.

As the social worker stood up to leave, Ms. C. asked if she would like to see Tommy's room: "I painted it myself." Standing in the doorway looking at the collection of toys surrounding the empty crib, the social worker sensed that this invitation was Ms. C.'s way of sharing her feelings of loss and emptiness. The worker exclaimed, "It's so empty without him!" For the first time this session Ms. C. looked directly at the social worker and her eyes filled with tears. The worker said, "I can see how much it hurts to be without him. If we can work together, I'm sure he will be able to come home again."

On the second home visit, the elevators in the housing project where Ms. C. lived were broken and the social worker had to climb twelve flights of stairs on a steamy summer day. By the time she arrived at Ms. C.'s door, she was breathless and trembling, not only from the unaccustomed exertion but also from fears generated by newspaper and television stories of muggings and stabbings in the project. Ms. C. greeted the worker, and, after looking her over for a moment, said, "You'd better sit down and have a cool drink!" Here was Ms. C.'s turn to "feed" the worker, who was touched by Ms. C.'s capacity for concern for her—a strength she believed could be mobilized to help Ms. C. in her mothering of Tommy.

During ensuing discussion, Ms. C. recalled growing up in a high-rise building with no elevators. Because her parents fought a lot she often sought sanctuary in her grandmother's apartment.

Ms. C.: She was strict but you always knew where you stood with her.

Worker: It sounds like you could count on her.

Ms. C.: Yes, not like my dad. We never even knew if he was coming home at night or if he would just start whipping us because he felt like it. Mom used to leave sometimes just so he wouldn't start beating up on her, too.

Worker: So there was nobody there to protect you?

Ms. C.: Not unless I could run to my grandmother's.

With the social worker's encouragement, Ms. C. went on to describe several memories of her grandmother. With great affection she recalled getting dressed up on Sundays to go to church. The grandmother loved to sing hymns in a very loud voice, and Ms. C. would stand by her side, swaying back and forth as she leaned against her leg and hummed along.

Worker: When you were with your grandmother you could feel good about yourself. You knew she really cared.

Ms. C.: I often used to think about her when things got bad after she passed. I'd think about her up in heaven singing with the angels and looking down on me.

When the social worker telephoned the following week to confirm the time of her next home visit, Ms. C. responded in a flat tone and said she was too tired to straighten up the apartment and would rather cancel the appointment. The social worker speculated that the sad feelings Ms. C. had experienced during the previous session might have precipitated some depression. The worker asked, "Do you think your not wanting me to come today could also have to do with all the memories we talked about last time?" Ms. C. said that she had spent a good part of the day after the last interview in bed and she didn't want to go through that again this week. The worker responded, "I think that you are so used to dealing with all your sad feelings by yourself that you are afraid to try it any other way. I would like to come today even though you don't want to talk to me. If you still feel the same way after we have talked a little, you can tell me and I will leave."

By the time the social worker arrived, Ms. C. had neatened the apartment. Again, she sat at the opposite end of the couch from the social worker. There was an awkward silence during which the worker pondered about how to reconnect with Ms. C. Then, almost imperceptibly, Ms. C. began to rock back and forth, singing softly to herself. At first the worker was unsure of the meaning of this behavior, and she wondered fleetingly if Ms. C. might be hallucinating. But as Ms. C.'s voice grew stronger, the worker recognized a hymn from her own childhood. Trusting her intuition that Ms. C. was trying to recapture the image of the good grandmother who had loved and protected her, the worker responded by singing softly. Ms. C.'s face lit up, and at the end of the next chorus of the duet, she stopped and said that she had found some photographs of her grandmother that morning and wanted to show them to the worker. She recalled happy memories about the things they had done together.

The visit ended with Ms. C. informing the social worker that she had made a medication follow-up appointment with the psychiatrist. She asked if she could come to see the social worker on the same day. As the worker confirmed the appointment, she realized that Ms. C. was sitting next to her on the couch. She had moved closer in order to be able to share with the worker the photographs of her grandmother.

In this case we see the value of focusing on ego relatedness in the initial engagement phase of intervention with the involuntary client. Consistently, the social worker sought out and attempted contact with the part of Ms. C. that, through the language of action, was asking for assistance. As the social worker prepared to meet Ms. C. for the first time, she achieved some empathic identification with her by tuning in to mental images generated by information received from collaterals. Her capacity to reflect quietly on the range and meaning of her apprehensive feelings fostered a primary therapeutic preoccupation that prepared her to offer Ms. C. a facilitating clinical environment. Her observations of Ms. C. and Tommy helped the worker gauge the parameters of optimal closeness and distance and, then, to arrange the interview in ways that would not threaten Ms. C. excessively.

The social worker conceptualized Ms. C.'s angry demeanor as a defensive posture that protected a frightened, vulnerable person. Frequently, it was as though the social worker were speaking into the void of Ms. C.'s angry silence. But because Ms. C. did not flee, this silence became an aspect of the potential space between them into which the social worker could place her own ideas about what Ms. C. might be experiencing. The worker worded her interventions in tentative, exploratory terms. These interventions were akin to what Bollas (1989) calls "musings" that the client can consider, agree, or disagree with, thus opening the possibility of dialogue. These musings serve a dual function: they demonstrate to the client the clinician's therapeutic preoccupation and efforts to understand; and they model for the client the process of reflecting upon one's own mental life.

To tune in to and make clinical use of internal associations requires that the clinician view and treat him- or herself as a subject in the treatment (Bollas 1989). The clinician learns to trust that his or her feelings and associations may be aspects of a fundamental ego relatedness to the client's inner experience. Especially in work with troubled clients whose vulnerabilities stem from early trauma and deprivation, the clinician can expect very strong feelings to surface. These feelings, often the result of projections and projective identifications designed to convey in feelings what the client cannot get into words, challenge the clinician's capacity to contain and metabolize intense affects. It is important for the clinician to have gained enough comfort with the full range of human affects to be able to treat these intense feelings as objects of contemplation rather than as things of action (Werner and Kaplan 1963). Ms. C.'s social worker, for example, felt but resisted the urge to comfort Tommy, or to tell Ms. C. to do so, when she first witnessed their physical estrangement in the emergency room cubicle. Rather than try to repair their relationship prematurely, the worker used her feeling of urgency as a possible signal of the depth of neediness that made Ms. C. keep a defensive distance. At other points in her work with Ms. C., the social worker experienced but suppressed powerful impulses to put her arms around her and comfort her, literally. While there may be instances where literal "holding" is indicated, to do so impulsively and in the absence of a compelling clinical rationale can lead to an unhelpful reparenting posture that can be more infantilizing than growth-promoting. As noted in Chapter 3, Winnicott deplored the conception of his work as professionalized kindness or reparenting and believed that clients needed to develop the capacity to use the clinical relationship symbolically rather than literally.

Clinicians working with reluctant or withholding clients need to have developed a capacity to be alone and to make productive use of their resulting inner states. Here, the social worker used silence as a time to turn inside to gather clues about what Ms. C. might be experiencing from her own feelings and fantasies. By tolerating Ms. C.'s attempts to shut her out—to leave her alone—the social worker demonstrated that it is possible to be alone in the presence of someone; and that this can be a useful relational medium.

In the case of Ms. C., it is easy to see the ways in which social and environmental factors can shape and perpetuate intrapsychic and interpersonal vulnerabilities. The holding environment for Ms. C.'s entire family was insecure, and self-esteem and feelings of competence were compromised across generations by insufficient socioeconomic provision, inadequate housing, and, because they were African-American, by institutionalized racism and oppression. Clinical assessment and intervention should include advocacy, collaboration with other social resources, and, where needed, the provision of concrete services to shore up the external holding environment so that ego relatedness can develop.

Difficulties with Drive and Impulse

Winnicott (1958) asserted that instinctual impulses arising from body experience can only be useful to the infant as a means of affirming the true self when experienced in a matrix of ego relatedness. In the comfortable, relaxed "unintegrated" state resulting from being alone in the caregiver's presence, "the stage is set for an id experience. In the course of time there arrives a sensation or an impulse. In this setting the sensation or impulse will feel real and be truly a personal experience" (p. 34). Here Winnicott suggests that, in the safe context of ego relatedness, the arising id impulse will strengthen rather than disrupt the ego. When the capacity to be alone has been compromised either through earlier relational disturbances or current trauma, sexual and aggressive impulses can disrupt internal continuity and threaten previously dependable ego defenses.

> Bob, a 19-year-old student, came to the college counseling service in a state of great anxiety. He was involved in a relationship that was providing him his first adult experience with sexual intimacy. While he was easily aroused, as soon as his girlfriend began to fondle his penis he experienced a feeling of "dread" and lost his erection. Exploration of his history revealed that during his childhood his mother had made a habit of bathing him and rubbing his back as a way of helping him get to sleep. If he got an erection, however, she scolded him and told him to "stop that." He developed increasing anxiety about going to bed and became panic-stricken if left alone before falling asleep. His distraught mother consulted a pediatrician who suggested a new bedtime routine: he was to bathe himself and was given music tapes to help him fall asleep. The anxiety abated until the adult experience of having a woman touch his penis resurfaced affects from the previous relationship in which sexual arousal had occurred in a context of overstimulation, loss of control, and punishment. In this instance the mother's disturbing response made her son's instinctual id experience feel dangerous and threatened his immature ego.

For clients whose ego functioning has been threatened in this manner, the clinician's aim is to provide a relational climate where such impulses can be considered from a developmental perspective and, thereby, employed in the service of psychosocial growth and integration.

Difficulties with the Capacity to be Alone

Early experience and current crisis combined to overwhelm the defenses of Mrs. O., a 57-year-old woman referred to a family service agency for treatment of a depression precipitated by learning of her husband's infidelity. She complained of despondency, lethargy, dizziness, loss of sexual drive, feelings of disgust toward her husband, and, most disturbing to her, an overriding fear of being alone. She worried that, if left alone too long, she might become ill and die before anyone found her. She talked of being "persecuted" by explicit mental images of her husband's sexual activities with his paramour. The fragility of her defenses and the corresponding fluidity between her mental and physical self-experience were expressed by fears that her brain would explode and by an extreme dizziness after bowel movements, the latter a symptom for which no physiological cause could be found. To the social worker, these intense feelings appeared to be "unbearable agonies," described by Winnicott (1962a) as feelings of going to pieces, of a distorted relationship to the body, of disorientation.

Exploration of Mrs. O.'s history revealed severe separation difficulties. As a child, she could not be left alone with a babysitter due to overwhelming feelings of panic and a conviction that she would never see her mother again. Beginning school at age 6, she was torn screaming from her mother's arms each day for the first year. Her mother's response was to weep helplessly; her father, in contrast, punished her for being "such a baby."

Also, an unusual family context helped explain the intensity of Mrs. O.'s disturbance then and its derivatives in her present situation. She was the youngest by nine years (the "baby") of six children in an Irish Catholic family. Several years prior to

Mrs. O.'s birth her mother had begun to offer the service of "laying out" the body of anyone who died in the closely knit neighborhood. As an infant and toddler, Mrs. O. accompanied and observed her mother as she went about her tasks, seemingly oblivious to their potential fearsome impact on her little daughter. Meanwhile, as her awareness grew, Mrs. O. became increasingly frightened by the sight of corpses and by the weeping of distraught relatives. She recalled fears of being spirited away by the "angel of death"—fears that were exacerbated by her mother's stern warnings that she must never walk on the wrong side of the road at night because half the road belonged to God and the other half to Satan, the latter always on the lookout for lost souls.

In the clinical relationship, Mrs. O.'s vulnerabilities expressed themselves from the beginning. She frequently told the social worker, a married woman, "All women are treacherous. They are like snakes in the grass!" Her reaction to the worker's efforts to help her reflect on the nature of her marriage prior to her husband's affair took the form of a dire prediction: "You wait and see! You think it won't happen to you, but it will. Your husband will be stolen away from you. There are women out there all the time just waiting to get a man in his weak moments. There isn't a man alive who can stand up to the temptation of a scheming woman." These predictions reminded the worker of Mrs. O.'s mother's warnings about the predatory Satan.

Beyond echoing an identification with her mother, these warnings seemed to express projections of Mrs. O.'s own jealous, acquisitive impulses and barely disguised her wish that the worker would suffer as she had—perhaps as a way of communicating to the worker the dreadful feelings that she could not get into words. To the worker it appeared that the mother's obliviousness to Mrs. O.'s terror had contributed to her pervasive sense of persecutory anxiety. This obliviousness could not be ascribed entirely to the mother's failure; it seems likely that Mrs. O. brought a constitutional predisposition to the situation that rendered her unusually sensitive to it. Whatever the combination of factors that precipitated her fear, Mrs. O. appeared to have been left psychologically alone prior to having internalized stable images of a reliable, soothing other and did not have a core experience of "going-on-being" in fearful situations. In the absence of this core of ego relatedness, impulses related to normal aggressive and destructive fantasies disrupted rather than strengthened her developing ego functions and defenses. As a result, splitting, projection, and projective identification emerged when she felt the threat of loss or abandonment. People, herself included, were all good or all bad—God or Satan. Rather than grow comfortable with her own aggressive impulses, she projected them onto other women—"snakes in the grass" who would rob her of her objects. In a world where the "angel of death" could come to seize her or those close to her, she could not tolerate being left alone. The separation panic originally aroused by her parents' absence was transferred to her husband and two daughters. For example, she could not tolerate her husband getting out of bed in the morning before she did, and she demanded that he call her from work several times a day. In addition, she recalled that she "almost had a nervous breakdown" when her older daughter left home to get married.

Mrs. O.'s case provides an illustration of the way vulnerabilities in ego relatedness compromise psychosocial development in later phases. Instinctual impulses in the anal phase stressed rather than strengthened her vulnerable ego. Because she experienced her bowel movements as a loss of part of her body, she suffered as a child from severe constipation. Her mother's response was to administer frequent laxatives and enemas. As an adult, Mrs. O. insisted that her husband administer the enemas. His compliance to this demand undoubtedly reflected his own unresolved issues.

Early difficulties also impaired Mrs. O.'s sexual functioning. Although she could become sexually aroused and find some enjoyment in intercourse, she experienced an acute sense of loss when her husband withdrew his penis. She became enraged when he "left" her after lovemaking by not talking as long as she expected or by falling asleep. Her competitive oedipal strivings were inhibited as well. A talented musician, she was forced to turn down a scholarship to a prestigious music school because accepting it would have meant facing the fearful prospect of moving to a distant city. As a music teacher, she feared retaliation from her female colleagues should she become more successful than they were. Similarly, she feared surpassing her teacher, also a woman, because it would mean she would have to move on to another.

Predictably, Mrs. O.'s separation difficulties and their derivatives manifested quickly in the clinical relationship. She had difficulty leaving the office at the end of each session and soon began making frequent between-session telephone calls to the social worker. To stabilize the clinical holding environment, the worker set time limits for ending each session and established a schedule of specific times she could be reached for brief phone contact between appointments. To foster ego relatedness and demonstrate her empathy for Mrs. O.'s struggles, the worker made statements reflecting her understanding of how frightening it was for her to leave. Mrs. O. responded with tearful gratitude that the worker could understand rather than react angrily to her "clinginess." Gradually, as ego relatedness stabilized, Mrs. O.'s projection of her problems onto her husband dissipated and she began to be able to reflect rather than act upon her intense affects. She could begin to consider how her desperate demands on her husband contributed to his infidelity, and they began to renegotiate their relationship toward greater tolerance for autonomy.

Interestingly, Mrs. O. confessed to the social worker that, early in the treatment process, she could not bring herself to dispose of the tissues she used in the session and that she also took home paper towels she had used in the bathroom adjacent to the office. Only a great act of will enabled her eventually to dispose of these items later. Mrs. O. seemed, at least initially, to need these concrete objects to sustain a sense of connection to the worker. As yet unable to internalize the therapist's soothing presence in a way that permitted her to soothe herself, she appeared to employ these items as transitional objects. In using transitional objects, Mrs. O. was crossing the bridge between ego relatedness and object relatedness. Winnicott (1953) believed that this journey is a necessary step in healthy development and represents a creative way for the person to be alone in the absence—as well as in the presence—of another.

In summary, ego relatedness is the primary sense of mutuality that develops between infants and their caregivers when an adequate holding environment has provided a sense of going-on-being. Unencumbered by overwhelming fears of personal annihilation and protected from internal and external impingements, the infant can experience unintegration—the safe, relaxed feeling of not having to work toward ego integration because the caregivers' reliable support can be taken for granted. In these periods of unintegration, normally arising instinctual impulses—part of the psychophysiologically alive true self—can strengthen rather than disrupt the development of ego functions and defenses. In these periods, the infant learns to be alone with his or her internal life while in the benign, nonintrusive presence of a reliable other. As cognitive and emotional development proceeds, the next item on the developmental agenda is internalization of a capacity to be alone in the absence of someone. This achievement is potentiated by the transitional process, typically expressed in Western culture by the attachment to transitional objects and phenomena.

In Winnicottian social work, this developmental process is viewed as a metaphor for the therapeutic relationship. A sufficient, supportive clinical holding environment fosters the development of ego relatedness between client and worker. As the client experiences the safety of the clinical context and the nonintrusive reliability of the clinician, he or she experiences a benign regression to dependence and develops the capacity to relax and "be alone" in the worker's presence. This capacity then makes possible object relating and, eventually, the use of the new object as a resource for achieving self–object differentiation and consolidating ego structuralization. The bridge between ego relatedness and object relatedness is the transitional process, some clinical manifestations of which we examine in the following chapter.

6

THE TRANSITIONAL
PROCESS

A 17-year-old high school senior came in for her weekly appointment at the school guidance office and surprised the social worker by pulling out a Polaroid camera and asking if she could photograph him. Quickly she took two pictures, handing one to the worker and putting the other in her purse. When asked about this behavior, she thought a moment before saying, "Even though we've been talking for several months now, sometimes I forget what you look like. I like the idea of having you along with me so I can remember when I need to."

At a college counseling service, an 18-year-old freshman who was having difficulty adjusting to living away from home recalled how upsetting it had been for him at age 10 when his family moved to a new city. Asked to reflect on his upset, he was surprised and embarrassed when he choked up with tears in conjunction with a memory that his mother had thrown out a favorite stuffed rabbit at that time. "Sometimes I still wish I had that rabbit," he said. "He was my good buddy."

At a family agency, a middle-aged mother of four grown children came in for help with her distress about a recent substantial weight gain and her inability to adhere to a diet prescribed by her doctor. In the second month of treatment, she began a session by saying, "Let me tell you about the weirdest dream I had last night. Telling you makes me feel a little silly, but here goes. A nice older man—not my father, but it sort of felt like that—came up to me and said, 'What would make you happy?' I replied without thinking, 'All the food I want and my teddy.'" Inquiry about what she thought the dream meant led to a memory of her fierce childhood attachment to a teddy bear and her father's insistence that she give it up when she turned 6. Her recollection was that, after her sixth birthday, the teddy bear "just disappeared." She was shocked at the intensity of her anger and sadness as she remembered not only her father's rigidity but her mother's compliance with his wishes that she give up the toy and "stop being a baby."

At a community mental health agency, a man with schizophrenia, despite having had the same weekly appointment day and time for several years, insisted that the social worker give him an appointment card on which she noted the time of their next meeting at the end of each session.

Winnicott's concept of transitional objects and phenomena, indisputably his most well-known contribution to psychoanalytic developmental theory, provides a framework for understanding the curious behaviors described in these vignettes. Andre Green (1978) notes that when Winnicott formulated the transitional object concept, he merely noticed "what had been escaping everyone's attention" and, in so doing, had "done nothing but discover the obvious" (p. 179). Winnicott, in other words, discovered an idea that was waiting to be found and, as in the process he so artfully described in his classic 1953 paper, he "created" it for our use in understanding a crucial segment of development.

With the attainment of ego relatedness, the infant is able to internalize the caregiver-as-environment and experiences a sense of oneness with her. At this stage, the introject is one of the caregiver as process rather than as object. Gradually, however, as the caregiver de-adapts her ministrations in synchrony with her infant's capacity to become more consistently self-regulating, the infant begins to experience this environment-mother as outside and to have a sense of difference from her. The dawning awareness of separateness prompts the infant to reach into the inanimate environment for some symbolic substitute for maternal care that tastes, feels, or smells like the caregiver. Winnicott believed the child's first true creative act to be the transformation of such an object into a symbol of maternal presence. The object *stands* for maternal care, but only because the child has made it happen.

Paradoxically, the child has appropriated something already in existence, but has "created" it anew by giving it personal meaning. By symbolizing the caregiver in this way, the infant has paved the way for what Winnicott called object relating. In Winnicott's idiosyncratic language, object relating refers to the infant's experience of the caregiver as a subjective object—one that, although having a "real" existence in the world, carries a reality unique to the baby's creative construction of her. Winnicott believed that the transitional object enabled the infant to make the transition from ego relatedness—that is, relatedness to caregiver-as-environment—to relatedness to the caregiver as a separate, yet personally constructed or subjectively conceived object.

As described in Chapter 2, transitional objects and phenomena inaugurate the capacity for illusion. With illusion, the developing child can play with ideas—can make one thing (a blanket or stuffed toy) stand for something else (a caregiver). This early capacity unfolds into a larger capacity for imagination, dreaming, and reverie. In later development, this capacity fosters empathy—the ability to play with the idea of being another while simultaneously being aware that one is not. Empathy is part of the "potential space" of clinical work—an intersubjective state, mutually created by client and clinician, in which meanings can be played with, puzzled about, reflected upon.

Just as the infant in the caregiver's absence turns to a transitional object to symbolize the maternal function, the client may at some point find a way to symbolize the soothing, facilitating clinical function. This phenomenon is a positive sign in treatment, suggesting that the client has taken a step in making the clinician his or her own—that is, a subjective object. In clinical work we see many people whose capacity for transitional relatedness has been compromised by various forms of environmental deprivation and associated developmental vulnerabilities. Clinicians need to be alert, therefore, to the junctures in intervention when clients begin to develop this capacity. Sometimes it becomes clear that we become transitional "objects" for clients; they may need to telephone between appointments, if only to hear a voice on the answering machine, in order to activate a self-soothing capacity. A child's request to take home a favorite toy from the playroom may indicate a struggle to symbolize the clinician between appointments. An appointment card provided at the end of a session can be transitional, serving as a concrete symbol of the clinician's reliability and constancy. An appreciation of the developmental importance of transitional relatedness can inform clinical intervention ranging from parenting education, to case management, to insight-oriented psychotherapy.

PARENTING EDUCATION

Helping parents accept and welcome the child's attachment to transitional objects and phenomena can facilitate later developmental progress. Through widespread public education about the crucial importance of bonding and attachment to healthy psychosocial development and well-being, there is general recognition of the facilitative role that transitional relatedness plays. There are instances, nevertheless, when, for reasons rooted in their own upbringing, parents are conflicted about their children's attachments to objects and benefit from educative intervention.

Mrs. K., referred to a family agency by her pediatrician, was having difficulty dealing with her 15-month-old son's wakefulness at night. In the initial interview conducted with mother and child, the social worker found Jason to be a vigorous, happy, inquisitive toddler. Initially leaning against the mother's knee, he gradually ventured out to explore the office and examine some toys offered by the worker. Periodically he scuttled back to the mother, demanding to be picked up. At other times he appeared to comfort himself by sucking his thumb and rubbing his baby blanket against his cheek.

The worker learned that, while Jason did not cry during his nocturnal awakenings, he called "mommy, mommy" repeatedly until she came. Asked what happened if she did not go to him, Mrs. K. said that she had not risked this; her husband believed that, should she not go, Jason would feel "abandoned and all alone in the world."

When the worker inquired about Jason's use of his baby blanket at night, she learned that he slept without it. Because Jason was so active, Mrs. K. worried that he might wrap it around his face and become unable to breathe. The worker resisted her urge to reassure Mrs. K. that would not happen and, rather, wondered aloud about where such a fear might have come from. Mrs. K. responded by recounting a long list of warnings passed on to her by her mother about dangers to avoid—suffocation among them—in child rearing. As Mrs. K.'s story unfolded, it emerged that her mother had spent her adolescence in a concentration camp. While she rarely spoke directly of this experience, she lived in terror of losing any of her family, and, during Mrs. K.'s childhood, compulsively checked on her whereabouts and safety. Once the origins of Mrs. K.'s fears were explored and discussed, she began to leave Jason's blanket with him at night. Almost immediately, he stopped calling for her and slept through the night.

Jason, developing normally and ready to use his baby blanket as a tool to help him be psychologically alone in his mother's absence, met an impediment in his mother's fears. That he called to her at night is not surprising; sleep for children represents a separation, and transitional objects are most likely to be used while the children are falling asleep (Winnicott 1953). The social worker's intervention, based on a knowledge of the developmental importance of the transitional process, cleared the path for Jason to make use of his capacity for illusion in the service of self-soothing.

Sleeping problems also troubled Alex, 12 years old, who was referred to a child guidance clinic by a family physician. Alex's parents reported that for the past three months he could fall asleep only if permitted to sleep on the floor in their bedroom or if one of them lay down with him in his room. In recounting Alex's history, the parents noted that there were also periods in his earlier life when he could not fall asleep alone. Exploration revealed that Alex's father could not bear to hear him cry as an infant. When he whimpered in the night, the father would rush to soothe him by picking him up and rocking him on his shoulder. The parents noted that Alex never did develop an attachment to a transitional object.

At age 4, Alex began having frightening dreams from which he woke in a panicky state. To prevent this, the father began sleeping beside Alex so that he could awake him as soon as he detected the agitation that he believed signaled the beginning of a nightmare. It appeared to the clinician that the father's over-availability had interfered with Alex's capacity to find self-soothing through transitional objects and phenomena and left him unprepared to cope by himself with frightening impulses, and their associated fantasies and dreams, aroused during the oedipal period. During the resurgence of these impulses that accompanied puberty, Alex had to revert to the literal human object for the experience of comfort and safety. The facilitation of the use of transitional objects can be particularly important, especially in Western cultures where children are expected to sleep alone from a very early age. (Further discussion of cultural variation in transitional object use appears in Chapter 9.)

CASE MANAGEMENT

Although a considerable literature has reported the application of the transitional object concept to psychoanalytically oriented psychotherapy (see Grolnick and Barkin 1978, Horton et al. 1988), very little has been written about its application to case management in nonpsychotherapeutic settings. Especially during periods of crisis or other upheaval in people's lives, an appreciation of the centrality of their attachments to transitional objects and phenomena can be crucial to successful intervention in a wide variety of service systems.

Winnicott believed that transitional relatedness, although originating in infancy, remains active throughout the life cycle and can be key in designing facilitating interventions at any point. Comstock (1981), for example, researched the value to elderly nursing home residents of being able to keep pictures and other transitional objects in their rooms. Not surprisingly, she found that being able to keep treasured mementos in their rooms smoothed their adjustment to nursing home life. Often, transitional relatedness constitutes a primary dynamic for elderly people who have sustained multiple personal losses and face further disruption to the continuity of their lives.

Mr. W., an 85-year-old widower, was referred by his family physician to the social service department of a geriatric hospital. Despite increasing abdominal pain and difficulty eating, Mr. W. refused to be admitted to the hospital for diagnostic tests. He ignored pleas from neighbors and his doctor's warnings about the seriousness of his condition. When the hospital outreach social worker telephoned to ask if she might visit and discuss his situation, he hung up on her. Finally, Mr. W.'s son flew in from another state and, against his father's wishes, set up an appointment for the social worker to make a home visit.

When the social worker arrived, Mr. W. left the house through the back door and began working in his vegetable garden. He appeared distraught and weak, breathing heavily and leaning on his spade for support. Shadowing his every move was an equally frail old dog. From the son the social worker learned that Mr. W. had lived in his home for fifty years and insisted on remaining after his wife's death ten years ago. Each of his three married sons had offered him a home, but he did not want to leave his garden and beloved dog.

The social worker, also an avid gardener and dog lover, went out to the garden to introduce herself. Undeterred by his lack of response, she sat down on an upturned bucket and began talking to the dog. The animal was friendly and responsive to this attention. Eventually Mr. W. grunted and said, "He'll take plenty of petting." The social worker agreed, but noted: "He never takes his eyes off you, though. It looks like you two are inseparable."

"You'd better tell Dr. Smith that," Mr. W. retorted. "He thinks I can just up and go to the hospital and leave all this!" His gesture included the garden, the dog, and the house. "Nobody understands how much this means to me. If I lost it life would not be worth living."

During two subsequent home visits, the social worker learned that the garden represented a connection with Mr. W.'s deceased wife. The two of them had worked in it side by side for years. Now when he worked there he felt close to her and, in fact, carried on long "conversations" with her. After his retirement he had belonged to a garden club and with many of his friends, now dead, had enjoyed exchanging plant cuttings. Mr. W. was able to point out to the social worker which friend had contributed a prize rose bush or a clump of irises. Clearly the garden was his link to past nurturing relationships.

In addition, dogs had played an important role in Mr. W.'s life since childhood, when he had lived on an isolated farm where his dog was often his best friend. As the social worker viewed it, the idea of losing both his present "friend" and his garden set off unbearable anxieties associated with loss and alienation from his familiar holding environment. Her challenge was to find a way to preserve his sense of environmental continuity while making it possible for him to receive the needed medical attention. She devised a plan based on the transitional object concept to make his care possible.

First she convinced Mr. W.'s sons to supplement his insurance coverage so that he could be admitted to a private room. Next she convinced the hospital medical director to admit the dog. The director's reluctant agreement hinged on the condition that the dog sleep under the bed—not on it, as was his custom—and that the visiting sons would use the service elevator to smuggle the dog out for a walk twice a day. Mr. W.'s sons also agreed to stay in the house and tend the garden daily until his discharge. The social worker helped Mr. W. select a few prized potted plants to take to the hospital.

With these arrangements in place Mr. W. agreed to admission and subsequently underwent surgery to remove an intestinal obstruction. During his convalescence Mr. W.'s dog kept vigil, occasionally licking his hand. Throughout the hospitalization the social worker met regularly with the nursing staff, the physician, the physical therapist, and cleaning personnel to give them a chance to talk about their concerns about having a dog on the unit. These ranged from worries about post-operative infection in a non-sterile environment to apprehensions about retribution for violating public health regulations. While Mr. W. was grateful to his family and the staff, he credited his successful recovery to the dog: "I knew I had to pull through for him."

In this case, the social worker's creativity and willingness to challenge the sanctity of hospital rules and regulations eased Mr. W. through a disruptive late-life medical crisis. Her awareness of the importance of transitional relatedness enabled her to devise an intervention plan that preserved Mr. W.'s defenses against the potentially overwhelming anxiety that might have erupted had he been forced to leave his familiar milieu. The social worker first forged a relationship to the dog, setting up the context for Mr. W. to reach out to her. This strategy circumvented his considerable resistance so that a relational link between them could be formed. Rather than interpreting Mr. W.'s fears or trying to get him to make connections between his present distress and past losses, the social worker used the idea of transitional relatedness to manipulate the environment in a way that would preserve his sense of going-on-being. Although she did not explain Winnicott's concept of transitional objects to the hospital staff, its intuitive validity made her plan seem sensible and workable.

Another vignette illustrates how the transitional process remains meaningful until the end of life and can foster humanistic care of the dying.

Mrs. R., a 91-year-old widow, had managed for several years to remain in her own small house despite heart problems and severely impaired mobility. When her health failed acutely, she found it increasingly impossible to maintain her resolve to stay in her own home "until the end." When a home care worker found her at noon one day in bed, disoriented and malnourished, she arranged for Mrs. R.'s admission to a local hospital. Once her condition was stabilized, arrangements were made to move her to a small, rural nursing home on the outskirts of her home town.

Mrs. R., never a socially comfortable person, kept to herself and became withdrawn and depressed in her new setting. When her heart problems flared up and she appeared to be near death, she seemed oddly agitated and distraught in ways that she could not verbalize to the staff or to visiting family. One day a stray kitten wandered into the nursing home lobby where Mrs. R. happened to be sitting in her wheelchair. The kitten came over to her, and she brightened, petting him and talking soothingly. Fortunately the staff recognized her mood change and were flexible in permitting the kitten to take up residence in Mrs. R.'s room. She named the kitten and the two became inseparable. The animal became a focus for conversation with other residents and staff members.

The staff observed that Mrs. R. seemed much more at peace after the kitten's arrival. It was as though her new attachment was soothing and made it possible for her to accept the nursing home placement. When she died two months later, the staff seemed to understand intuitively that Mrs. R. had been able to use the kitten as an object that facilitated her transition to dying. This capacity to perceive and permit transitional relatedness became a pivotal component in the management of Mrs. R.'s care.

Beyond management, the transitional object concept can guide sensitive intervention with clients who, although in need of assistance, are not easily engaged. With Ms. C., the client discussed in Chapter 4 who burned her 2-year-old son's arm, the social worker's understanding of transitional objects and phenomena became the key to engaging Ms. C. in a productive relationship. In fact, transitional objects literally brought them together.

> When on the second home visit Ms. C. began rocking and singing to herself, the social worker recognized that the developing clinical relationship was evoking soothing memories of the "good" nurturing grandmother of Ms. C.'s childhood. The hymn was a transitional phenomenon, much like a lullaby, that Ms. C. could draw on as a source of comfort and evocative memory. When she and the social worker finished singing, Ms. C. brought out photographs of her grandmother—treasured transitional objects—the viewing of which required that Ms. C. and the social worker sit next to each other. With music and pictures, they discovered a shared intermediate area, or potential space, in which their engagement could be solidified and affirmed. This transitional process was pivotal in the development of trust that gradually allowed Ms. C. to relinquish her distant, hostile posture and reveal her vulnerability to the worker. The transitional process became another dimension of the holding environment of treatment that enabled Ms. C. to "hold" rather than abuse Tommy, who was eventually returned to her care.

THE TRANSITIONAL PROCESS IN ASSESSMENT AND INTERVENTION

In making assessments, it is important to determine whether or not a capacity for transitional relatedness has been achieved developmentally. Sometimes attachments that appear to serve a transitional function are, in fact, not truly transitional but act as literal "substitute objects" (Barkin 1978). Lacking a transitional meaning, these objects do not foster a capacity for illusion and fail to facilitate the internalization of a self-soothing capability that makes relinquishing them possible.

Such was the case with Ms. P., a 19-year-old single woman who was referred to a social worker who worked for her employee assistance plan. She made the initial call to the worker's home on Thanksgiving day and explained, between sobs, that her dog had been killed by a car that morning and that, as a result, she was feeling suicidal. Although she lived with a boyfriend and had a few friends, "Only the dog truly understood" her feelings: "When I was upset I would put my head on his tummy and tell him my troubles. He would lick away my tears."

While Ms. P. had difficulty accepting the reality that she could not be seen that afternoon, she did agree to an appointment for the next morning. She again telephoned the worker—this time at 3:00 A.M.—to report extreme agitation and obsessional thoughts about the dog that prevented her from falling asleep. She felt she could not disturb her boyfriend because he was tired of hearing about the dog and needed to get up and to go work the next morning.

During her appointment the next morning, Ms. P. recounted a history of chaotic relationships. Her father was alcoholic and had abandoned the family when she was 3 years old. Her mother had subsequently lived with a succession of men who were physically abusive to Ms. P. and her siblings. To escape this Ms. P. had run away from home at age 16 and eventually moved in with a man twice her age. She had left him six months previously to move in with her current boyfriend. Now she was thinking of quitting her job because her boss was too critical.

Ms. P. wanted the social worker to "make me feel better." She warned that this must be accomplished in three sessions—the company insurance plan provided for three full sessions, after which Ms. P. would be required to pay half the fee for subsequent appointments. When the worker suggested that three visits might not be sufficient, Ms. P. seemed perplexed and wanted him to waive the fee altogether.

Toward the end of this first interview, Ms. P. told the worker that she'd been thinking about going to the animal shelter that day to obtain another dog. The worker's decision to support this plan was based on his recognition that Ms. P.'s ego functioning was too impaired and stressed for her to sustain the clinical relationship past one session. She seemed not to have a capacity to tolerate her anxiety and delay gratification long enough to work collaboratively on her problems. Rather than a true transitional object that sponsored ego integration, the dog in this case was a substitute rather than a symbol for the missing caregiver. The need to replace the dog immediately suggests that, as an object, it had little relational meaning beyond that of need gratification. Ms. P. viewed the social worker similarly—he was to be a source of immediate gratification who would meet her demands unconditionally.

Clinically we also see clients who appear to have attained a capacity for transitional relatedness in early life but who, due to environmental deprivation or disturbance, regress to a pre-transitional mode of managing separation anxiety. Gaddini (1978) refers to pre-transitional attachments as "precursor objects," deriving from the time in infancy prior to the appearance of transitional objects when the baby employs thumbsucking, hair-stroking, or other uses of parts of his or her own or the caregiver's body for self-soothing. As parts of either the baby's own or the caregiver's body, such attachments are not "transitional" because they do not yet belong to the intermediate "potential space" between self and other. Although certain eating disorders have been conceptualized as a use of the body as a transitional object (Sugarman and Kurash 1982), we see many eating disorders, including some cases of obesity, as derivative of precursor attachments.

Such was the case with Mr. E., a 30-year-old man who was 150 pounds overweight and sought services at a community mental health clinic. Following a period of frequent bouts of hyperventilation and sleeplessness, he consulted the family doctor. The doctor referred him to counseling for these symptoms as well as for his obesity, a condition that was increasingly impairing his physical health. The social worker learned during the evaluation that Mr. E. was feeling "stuck" at home with his divorced mother and in his unchallenging job at a neighborhood grocery store. The more anxious he felt, the more he ate—"even when I'm not hungry; I just feel quieter when I'm eating."

Though he remembered little about his early years, family stories caricatured him as "the nicest boy—quiet, and never any trouble." He did have isolated memories, going back to age 5, of taking care of his father when he was "under the weather" from drinking too much. In fact, on two occasions when his mother was working the night shift as a nurse's aide, the little boy found his father passed out on the floor and bleeding from a fall. He not only called the police for help, he accompanied his father to the hospital in the ambulance. Mr. E. recalled feeling terrified by the lights and loud noise of the ambulance, sitting next to the stretcher with his eyes closed and his hands over his ears. He was both relieved and saddened by his parents' divorce when he was 8. The father subsequently moved across country and had seen his son only annually for several years.

Mr. E. quickly formed a working alliance with the social worker. By the end of the first six months, he had obtained a more interesting job and was taking a course toward completion of his high school diploma. He had also begun a medically supervised diet and lost 50 pounds. The counselor was surprised, therefore, when these apparent gains were followed by a regressive period during which Mr. E. began missing work so that he could watch television and eat, slowly regaining weight.

Exploration revealed that, with weight loss, Mr. E. had begun to feel more anxious. He recalled catching a reflection of himself in a store window and feeling disoriented and frightened. He noticed that his wrist bones were more pronounced, and his face seemed to be changing. Eating calmed these feelings, and he reported an odd sense of relief as he began to gain weight. When the counselor wondered if the weight served a protective function, his response was, "It makes me feel safe. I created it. It belongs to me alone." Asked to recall other things that made him feel safe, he was surprised to find himself thinking about a favorite blanket from childhood. His mother had teased him later that he was "never without it; you were either dragging it around or had it wrapped around you like a cape, pretending to be Superman." He had a specific memory about the end of this attachment. Home from the hospital after a period of detoxification, the father had begun to demand that he give up the blanket and stop being a "sissy." Only age 5, the boy still used the blanket while falling asleep. Although inconsolable without it, he had no choice but to watch helplessly as the father tore it into shreds and threw it away. Since it was during Mr. E.'s fifth year that he had begun to gain weight, the counselor mused with him that his weight might serve as something he could wrap around himself to preserve a sense of safety and invulnerability—a permanent, protective cape under his sole control that gave him the feeling of omnipotence that he imagined Superman to possess. This formulation seemed to be helpful to Mr. E. as he continued to work on issues related to his obesity and to his struggles about dependency.

As the social worker viewed it, when Mr. E. was forced to relinquish his blanket before he was ready to do so, he regressed to the oral gratification of eating for self-soothing. In his case, the resulting obesity assumed the sort of protective function usually served by transitional objects and phenomena. But because the weight was part of his body, it was more a precursor than a transitional object—it was not part of the transitional intermediate area of experiencing that fosters further development, but rather a regressive attachment that kept him "stuck" in a regressive, dependent posture. Once he began to use the worker as a transitional "object," he was able to work on understanding these issues and began to make changes in his situation. Subsequent bouts of anxiety and overeating could be taken up in terms of feeling frightened, alone, and needing to wrap his security "blanket" around himself again.

Clearly, symptoms like Mr. E.'s are multidetermined and can be neither explained nor altered solely on the basis of the type of formulation described above. The social worker's awareness of transitional relatedness as a developmental issue, however, did provide a way of thinking about his weight that became useful as a metaphor for understanding and talking about it. This idea helped Mr. E. appreciate that his current difficulties and behavior had meaning associated with unresolved earlier issues.

Winnicott (1953) noted that, although attachments to specific objects tend to disappear as children internalize a capacity for self-soothing and symbolization, "A need for a specific object or behavior pattern that started at a very early date may reappear at a later age when deprivation threatens" (p. 91). This idea leads naturally to a consideration of manifestations of transitional relatedness that appear at later periods of psychosocial development. Several authors, for example, have examined clinical implications of transitional relatedness in adolescence (Anderson 1978, Benson 1980, Downey 1978, Fox 1977). Applegate (1984) has connected transitional phenomena in adolescence to Blos's (1967) concept of adolescence as a "second individuation." Relating ego development in adolescence to the separation-individuation process of the first three years of life, Blos suggests that adolescent struggles around dependence and independence catalyze a normal regressive pull that involves "the re-experiencing of abandoned or partly abandoned ego states which had been either citadels of safety and security, or which once had constituted special ways of coping with stress" (p. 173). Among the citadels of safety and security in early childhood are transitional objects and phenomena, and adolescents may employ them as ways of coping with the demands, both instinctual and societal, for separation and independence. Viewing adolescence through this lens helps explain such perplexing behavior as overuse of the telephone, vegetative television watching, perpetual wearing of stereo headphones, and attachments to articles of clothing.

Similarly, when early development or difficult life circumstances have interfered with the capacity for transitional relatedness, the resulting vulnerabilities are likely to reappear at adolescence and frequently bring young people to clinical settings.

> John, an 18-year-old college freshman, sought treatment after his girlfriend ended their two-year relationship. After learning that she was dating someone else, he stopped studying and going to classes and was placed on academic probation. Increasingly he spent entire days in his room smoking marijuana and listening to music. A concerned classmate urged him to come to the college counseling service for help.
>
> John's initial posture was one of intensity and bravado. He sometimes paced in the office, gesticulating and swearing. He wondered how talking could help—it only stirred things up. "All I want to do is smoke dope and space out." Over several months his essential loneliness was revealed: he needed his girlfriend to feel "whole."
>
> Asked to talk more about the use of marijuana, he recounted vivid sensory images. He appeared transported in the office as he described the careful rituals related to "smoking," and he detailed various textural and olfactory sensations. "It's like I can lie back and get peaceful," he stated. "I'm warm and whole again. I blend into the music." Without this aid he felt tense, agitated, "As if I'm trying to find something I've lost—but I don't know what it is."
>
> The social worker's interventions focused on the affect hunger John experienced without marijuana and the illusion of soothing "wholeness" he captured with it. The contemporary event of losing his girlfriend appeared to revive earlier losses, longings, and disappointments. The eldest of six children, he recounted early school troubles and a sense of being "pushed aside" at home as each new sibling arrived. He recalled sitting outside his mother's room as a latency-age child, listening to her singing lullabies to the new baby and feeling oddly saddened

and comforted. Together, he and the therapist came to understand that the loss of the girlfriend made him feel similarly
"pushed aside," losing closeness to a nurturing person once
again.

John relaxed more in the office. Having taken some time off
from school, he re-entered and did well. He began to date a variety of young women, one of whom introduced him to Transcen-
dental Meditation. He began to practice this and enjoyed the
social relationships he made attending some college-sponsored
group meetings about meditation. The use of marijuana "went
away," as he put it, except at social occasions when it became
part of peer group experience.

John employed marijuana smoking as a way to recapture
an intermediate experience with elements of symbiotic merger. The "object" was not part of himself, yet it had many
soothing qualities reminiscent of maternal comfort. Kahne
(1967) indicates that transitional object use in later development occurs when there is a threat of separation from an
important contemporary object—in John's case, the "object"
was the girlfriend. Ritvo (1971) has indicated that in late adolescence, "marijuana and the psychedelic drugs are likely to
be used at times of great loneliness, object hunger, narcissistic wounds to the ego, that is, when preoedipal strivings
are intensified" (p. 259). For John, smoking marijuana was
a regressive return to orally derived self-soothing. Combining this with listening to music fostered further affective recollection of imagined idyllic reconnection with the nurturing mother.

The social worker's recognition of these behaviors as transitional phenomena conveyed respect for John's flounder-
ing attempts at self-soothing. A resulting sense of being understood seemed to promote trust in the therapist that enabled
John to look at the meaning of his actions and begin to
modify them. Subsequent employment of meditation as a
more integrative way to alter his consciousness reflected a
greater capacity for non-drug induced illusion and more con-

trolled adaptive regression (Shafii 1973). His membership in a peer group formed around this activity allowed for less ambivalently laden social relationships.

A very specific transitional object became the focus for treatment of another adolescent.

A handsome, shy 17-year-old high school senior, Roger came to a family agency following an acute depressive episode in which he mentioned to his sister that he had some suicidal thoughts. Previously a model student, Roger's school performance was slipping and he withdrew from friends. The parents, both lawyers, assumed he would go to college as his sister had. His depression worsened when a letter of acceptance came from a college in another state.

In initial interviews with the social worker, Roger was uneasy and silent. Gradually he began to share his "terror" of going away to school. With support he was able to convey this to the parents who, after a consultation with the worker, reluctantly agreed to his waiting a year before beginning college. In subsequent sessions with the social worker, he revealed his place in the family as his mother's confidant. He viewed the parents' relationship as formal and distant, believing that they had an unhappy marriage. He bought his mother inappropriate gifts and often went shopping with her. The father remained relatively uninvolved.

With the pressure off about college, Roger's mood improved. He began to talk about buying a car and shared detailed accounts of his search for "just the right one." He settled on a conservative sedan more suitable to an older adult than to an adolescent, and proudly showed his new acquisition to the worker. There ensued a preoccupation that consumed many treatment sessions. Roger's goal was to keep the car "perfect." He acquired every conceivable accessory and kept the car garaged to protect it on all but the sunniest days. His parents gave him rides to his part-time job during inclement weather, essentially colluding in his preoccupation with the illusion of automotive perfection.

In treatment the car became a symbol for Roger's struggles around separation-individuation. The car provided safe forays into the world beyond his parents and back again, in "good weather." Roger described peaceful times alone cleaning and polishing the car, or installing the latest gadget. The constant care required to preserve the car's perfection offered a focus for his concerns that seemed to deflect both internal separation fears and external demands that he move on. During this period Roger gave the social worker a beautifully crafted model car that he had assembled. Later in this phase, the worker gave Roger some newspaper articles about classic cars.

Roger's marked depressive reaction to a small dent in his car's fender provided an opportunity to work through the loss of the illusion of omnipotence. The dent symbolized the failure of his perfectionistic strivings and self-expectations. As he grieved the illusory "perfect" car, he began to tolerate and express more ambivalence toward his parents; he was particularly disillusioned that his mother could "let me go away" to college. Gradually he could look with the worker at how collusive family interactions around the car served to foster his dependency.

Roger's difficulties appeared to be aroused by the specter of separation from home. His "perfect" car, created by his customizing efforts, afforded him a transitional space—an illusion of the idealized relationship to a "perfect" caregiver that also symbolized a way to leave her. In treatment, he needed to share this transitional experience in detail and, through the metaphor of the car, he verbalized preoedipal longings and disappointments. Later, the ability to let the sedan go and purchase a sports car more appropriate to adolescent male phallic expressiveness heralded his readiness to move toward resolution of oedipal conflicts on his way to adulthood.

THE CLINICIAN AS TRANSITIONAL OBJECT

Noting the transitional function for some clients of his role as clinician, Winnicott (1962b) wrote, "In this position I have some of the characteristics of a transitional phenomenon, since although I represent the reality principle, and it is I who must keep an eye on the clock, I am nevertheless a subjective object for the patient" (p. 166). When the development of the transitional process is understood and fostered in the facilitating clinical partnership, the client moves toward a deepened capacity for reflective consideration of the complexity of his or her situation. This reflection occurs in the intermediate area or potential space between client and clinician. As the ability to retain a constant mental representation of the clinician as a beneficial new object grows, the client can increasingly experience phases of unintegration and is freed to play with a multiplicity of meanings. Through the vehicle of the transitional process, the client transports aspects of the supportive clinical holding environment inside. Tolpin (1971) suggests that this process occurs through transmuting internalization—that is, a taking in by the client of soothing functions of the clinician and the clinical setting and giving them the stamp of the client's own creative rendering. For the client, the resulting mental representation of the clinician is a mixture of qualities of the real clinician and the image of the clinician forged from the client's unique perceptions—an object, like the transitional object, that resides in the potential space between "me" and "non-me." This sequence is crucial, therefore, to the building of intrapsychic structure.

As the client comes to trust the holding qualities of the clinical setting and begins to employ the transitional process to render the clinician a reliable subjective object, the stage is set for a transformation in the therapeutic relationship through which the clinician becomes a usable, objective object for the client. To understand how this occurs, we turn to Winnicott's (1971e) conception of the developmental journey from object relating to object usage and its manifestations in clinical social work.

7

OBJECT RELATING
AND
OBJECT USE

With the help of the transitional process, the developing child moves to a new stage of relatedness and intrapsychic structuralization. This move, which enables the child to preserve aspects of the primary illusion, also sponsors his or her readiness to become adaptively disillusioned. For this disillusionment to be growth promoting, "everything hinges on the changeover from mother as a subjective object to an object objectively perceived; from seeing himself through the other, to seeing the other" (Phillips 1988, p. 130). When this transformation from object relating to object usage occurs, the client "feels contact has been made with something genuinely other that resists coercion" (p. 110)—a resistance that "affords him the definition of his own limits" (p. 109). And, as described in Chapter 2, Winnicott believed that establishing and testing these limits happens through aggression that is catalyzed both by the caregiver's inevitable failures and by the individual's own innate thrust toward self-object differentiation. If the "failures" are tolerably attuned to the child's evolving capacity to bear them, and if the caregiver can "survive" the aggression they arouse without retaliating, they can be used as opportunities for internalization and organization of distinct self and object images into enduring intrapsychic structure. This structural achievement includes development of the superego, as the child experiences anxiety and guilt about possibly "destructive" fantasies and impulses and gains a capacity for concern along with wishes to make reparation. Repeated experiences of this "benign circle" pave the way for interpersonal relationships characterized by the capacity to be self-sustaining alongside a capacity to be intimate with and concerned about others.

Clients who have not successfully navigated this process tend to persist in viewing important others in their lives, including the clinician, in subjective terms. To defend against anxieties associated with disillusionment—which, to them, may feel like abandonment and/or annihilation—they often employ such mechanisms as denial, projection, and projective identification to preserve the subjective object and resist taking in the reality that others are separate and, to some extent, beyond control. Indeed, clinical social work— especially with those clients whose backgrounds have exposed them to deprivation and retaliation in response to their normal assertive strivings—calls on clinicians to be accepting of aggression and clients' periodic need to "destroy" them as they test the helping relationship for its durability. Many clients have grown up in socioeconomic contexts where environmental deprivation made it difficult for caregivers to respond flexibly and adaptively to their normal assertive strivings. Rather than support their children's thrusts toward differentiation, some caregivers have retaliated through neglect and abuse, or have in more subtle ways socialized their children toward docility and compliance. Such responses foreclose the eventual development of a capacity to view others objectively and empathically, thus jeopardizing the development of a capacity for concern. Moreover, persistent retaliation against or frustration of nonhostile self-assertiveness may lead to a relational style dominated by hostile destructiveness and sadism (Parens 1979, Stechler and Halton 1987).

> Evelyn, an 18-year-old mother, brought her 6-month-old son Stephen for a well-baby visit. The pediatric clinic social worker saw Evelyn slapping Stephen's hands as he reached up to explore her face and to pull at her nose as they sat in the waiting room. When later invited to tell the worker how she felt when Stephen behaved this way, Evelyn responded angrily, "He's got to learn he can't go around pushing people in the face." She had no idea that this was her son's way of getting to know her and to explore the limits of his own and others' worlds. The likelihood is that, left unaddressed, this retaliation to his assertive explorations would subdue healthy assertion and model hostile-aggressive interactions.

With some clients, social workers may need to be ready for repeated tests of their ability to "survive without retaliating," while preserving the benign support of a firm holding environment. In some instances, detecting how the worker is being tested and otherwise "used" may be difficult and requires access to and reflective examination of strong countertransference feelings. As Bollas (1987) notes, signs of a shift from object relating to object usage can often be detected only through their appearance in the internal experience of the clinician. Turning to countertransference feelings, we consider how we feel used: Do we feel attacked, abandoned, depleted, smothered, or subject to impervious indifference? All these states may represent aspects of the client's experience with important objects that he or she cannot get into words. Applying this concept to analysis, Bollas (1987) suggests that "The infant element in the adult patient speaks to the analyst through that sort of object usage that is best 'seen' through the analyst's countertransference. The infant within the adult person cannot find a voice, however, unless the clinician allows the patient to affect him, and this inevitably means that the analyst must become disturbed by the patient" (p. 204). To weather such disturbance, the social worker needs the time and support to reflect on the impact and meaning of the strong subjective states aroused in the process of beginning to be "used." Often crucial tests occur during beginning contacts.

Mr. F., a stocky, muscular construction worker, was mandated by the court to seek social work services after having been reported for child abuse by a teacher at his son's school. Five-year-old Robbie had come to school repeatedly with large welts and bruises on his arms and legs. Mr. F. was outraged by this interference in his life and defended his right to "discipline" his son just as his father had disciplined him—with a leather belt. "You don't waste your breath talking to kids. That's not what they understand. You *show* them!" He rebuffed the social worker's efforts to get to know him, declaring that "I've been out earning a living since I was 12 years old. Nobody is going to tell me how to run my life." Observing father and son together, the worker noted a strong attachment. But Mr. F. appeared uncomfortable with Robbie's affectionate hugs and requests to sit on his lap, viewing such behavior as evidence that Robbie could turn into a "sissy."

For the first few weeks of the court-ordered treatment, Mr. F. telephoned at the last moment to change his appointment time, giving the social worker a list of alternative times when he could fit her into his schedule. When they did meet he frequently criticized her manner of dress, the way she spoke, and the "namby-pamby" way he imagined she thought children should be reared. Seeking consultation when her own hurt and angry feelings began to feel unmanageable, the worker was able to tolerate his provocative behavior without striking back. Over and over she verbally acknowledged Mr. F.'s rage and resentment while also making it clear that the court required that they meet so they could get some understanding of why he periodically lost control and injured Robbie. Although he frequently called her disparaging names over the phone, she maintained a professional demeanor, greeting him in a respectful, friendly manner. She was able to do this because she made it a point to take time before each session to reflect on the probable meaning of his angry attacks. She surmised that he belittled her in the way he felt belittled by having to come for help. In addition, she scheduled a few minutes after each session to have a cup of tea and replenish herself as she reflected on her upset feelings as possible indicators of the way she was being "used" by Mr. F. This vigil of her internal life made it possible for the worker to survive the long period of testing of her durability as well as Mr. F.'s projection onto her of his unacknowledged, awkward "namby-pamby" self.

The serendipitous discovery of a mutual interest provided the transitional bridge into a potential space where Mr. F. and the worker could meet on more neutral territory. In one session, Mr. F. happened to mention his long-standing interest in opera— also an interest of the worker's. She began to make use of their shared interest to give voice to themes of loss, betrayal, disappointment, and family conflicts as portrayed in various operas. Initially, Mr. F. took center stage in these discussions, using the worker as an audience to lengthy monologues designed to strut his superior operatic knowledge and further belittle her. But one day during a discussion of Othello's tragic inability to realize how much Desdemona loved him and of his vulnerability to Iago's destructive influence, the worker remarked that Mr. F. was a lot like Othello—his own insecurities made it impossible for him to love to his full capacity. Mr. F.'s eyes filled with tears; then he became furious, loudly proclaiming that he knew who he was and didn't need the worker to tell him what he was feeling. The worker noted how uncomfortable he found it to share his sad feelings with her. She then reminded him how moving it was to see Othello weep so inconsolably after he killed Desdemona and how much it would take away from the opera were he unable to show this anguish. This intervention served to recognize and legitimate the value of Mr. F.'s feelings of sadness and vulnerability, while gently acknowledging the defensive nature of his physical bravado. He became calmer after this session and began to talk more about himself and to share affects other than derisive anger.

When anger did reappear, he could begin to address it more reflectively. After one particularly difficult weekend with Robbie, he admitted feeling utter helplessness, then rage, when his son did not do as he was told immediately. His reaction was that his son's mild non-compliance offered proof that Robbie had no respect for Mr. F.'s authority and saw him as a "wimp." When asked to talk about how he was disciplined as a child, Mr. F. told the worker that he never dared question his parents' authority because doing so resulted quickly in a whipping with father's belt. He recalled fantasies of being big and strong enough to overpower his father at these times. After one severe beating he wrote, "When I grow up I am going to buy a gun and kill you," and then put the note inside a bottle and buried it in the back yard. As he talked more about his impotent anger as a child, Mr. F. began to see the connections between this anger and his need to be in control of the worker. He cried as he recognized that he was doing to Robbie, and figuratively to the worker, what had so terrified him as a child.

This vignette offers a clear illustration of the movement from treating the clinician as a subjective object—one shaped by projections of unacknowledged aspects of self—to viewing her as an external object who could become part of his shared reality and, therefore, available for use in the service of self-exploration. The worker recognized in Mr. F.'s love of opera a manifestation of a capacity for transitional relatedness. She then drew on this imaginative capacity to make way for a "potential space" between them in which Mr. F. could contact and express carefully hidden vulnerable feelings. As he became more comfortable with these feelings, he became better able to tolerate them in Robbie. The worker's patient survival of Mr. F.'s early attacks assured him that she could survive the intensity of his feelings. He moved from using her as an object of abuse, to using her as an audience for his display of expertise about opera, to an eventual use of her as a collaborative partner in exploring issues of vulnerability and dependency.

In other instances, both early experience and later life choices have compromised the move from viewing others as subjectively conceived to seeing them as separate, self-regulating others.

Mrs. Q., a 62-year-old widow, came to a family service agency asking for help with unbearable feelings of grief and depression following her husband's death six months earlier. Exploration of Mrs. Q.'s experience of her husband's death revealed that her grief was dominated by rage that she had no control over his "leaving" her. During the thirty-six years of their marriage they had done everything together and, because of the closeness of their relationship, had decided not to have children. As Mrs. Q. described their day-to-day life it became apparent that they did not treat each other as separate psychological entities. Mr. Q. dictated his wife's hair color and style while she chose his clothes. Neither could tolerate a difference of opinion: "I always knew what he wanted. We were so close he felt like my skin. I don't know who I am without him!"

Mrs. Q. had moved directly from her mother's home into marriage. As she described it, "I've never had to think for myself in my life. First my mother told me what to do and then my husband took over." Now she bitterly resented having to do things by herself. Even pleasurable activities became reminders that she was "forced" to be alone. She felt physically ill when alone in bed and was unable to sleep without tranquilizers.

Mrs. Q.'s account of her history suggested that her mother had difficulty adapting to her daughter's natural moves toward independence. She dressed Mrs. Q. in long frilly dresses that impeded her learning to walk, and she kept her out of school until age 7. Mrs. Q. was not permitted to choose her own clothes, hair style, or foods. If she did not return immediately from school her mother accused her of "killing" her with worry. This overconcern persisted into adulthood. Once after Mrs. Q. was married and her mother could not reach her by telephone she arrived at her home with the police. Throughout her life

Mrs. Q. struggled with a wish to murder her mother so she could be free, yet the fear that her wish would come true paralyzed her with guilt.

In the transference, Mrs. Q. controlled early sessions by loud wailing that prevented any meaningful communication. She frequently called the social worker between sessions to change her appointment because she had decided to have her hair or her nails done. If she could not sleep she would call the agency and be surprised that the worker was not there and would not be returning her call that evening. In the countertransference, the worker's experience of being with Mrs. Q. was that she was trying to hold a kicking, screaming child in the throes of a temper tantrum. In time it became clearer that Mrs. Q.'s loud wails were ruthless attacks on the worker—attacks that the worker handled empathically but firmly. Leaning forward in her chair, the worker would say, "Mrs. Q., I am going to interrupt you so that you can hear what I have to say. I know you cannot take me in when you are crying so loudly." In the midst of one particularly stormy session Mrs. Q. cried out, "I don't know how you can stand my grief!" She appeared surprised to hear that the worker was not feeling grief-stricken, but was feeling relatively calm. After six weeks of twice weekly sessions, Mrs. Q. came in with a small bunch of flowers: "I thought I'd bring in something to cheer you up today since I'm always so miserable to be with." In fact, the worker liked Mrs. Q. and was able not only to thank her but to state genuinely that she did not find Mrs. Q. miserable to be with. This session marked a turning point in Mrs. Q.'s capacity to perceive the worker as a distinct person. She began to notice and comment on her hair style, manner of dress, and tone of voice. Outside the sessions Mrs. Q. became involved in some volunteer work and in other ways became less focused on her own difficulties.

The social worker's capacity to "survive" Mrs. Q.'s "attacks," disguised as intense grief, helped establish boundaries to the relationship that allowed Mrs. Q. to experience the worker and herself as distinct entities. Apparently neither Mrs. Q.'s mother nor her husband could tolerate her assertive efforts to differentiate, and the frustration of these strivings led to intense, even murderous, hostile-aggressive impulses. The worker's capacity to use her countertransference to identify, weather, and set some limits on the hostile aggression in Mrs. Q.'s behavior led to Mrs. Q.'s wishes to make reparation for the "misery" she inflicted. Learning that the worker did not find her "miserable to be with"—that the worker was not just a repository of her own projections—helped Mrs. Q. become aware of the worker's distinct attributes. From this process evolved a capacity for concern and a wish to contribute to others.

Mr. F.'s and Mrs. Q.'s early displays of hostile-aggressive testing were somewhat unusual, probably related to their overall style of defense. More typically it is only when a sense of safety and trust finds solid footing in a secure clinical holding environment and ego relatedness with the clinician is established that clients can begin to risk testing the clinician's durability.

Such was the case with Ms. J., a 23-year-old nurse who came to a community mental health clinic with the complaint of "being scared to death." Her symptoms, triggered by her boyfriend's pressure to become engaged, included colitis, difficulty falling asleep, fear of the dark, loss of appetite, panic attacks during which she feared dying from a heart attack, and a terror of going crazy.

The second child in an Irish Catholic family of four children, Ms. J. reported earlier episodes of colitis and acute anxiety, usually associated with separations. She recalled, for example, that she had trouble separating from her mother as a toddler and was the only one of the children who could not tolerate being left with a baby sitter when her mother went off to work. She viewed herself as an over-functioning child who, due to her mother's emotional fragility and her father's detachment, took over much of the care of the house and her younger siblings. Her mother took great pride in her little girl's capacity to care for the family and Ms. J. came to value herself as one who met the needs of others regardless of the personal cost. As an adolescent and young adult, Ms. J. received uneven support and mixed messages from her parents. Although they encouraged her to go to the movies with friends, for example, the absence of a regular allowance made it impossible to meet the condition that she pay for such entertainments out of her own pocket. At age 16 she began working during the summers in order to "buy some independence," and was able to save enough money to begin college. Though she did well academically, close relationships proved troublesome. Not until Mark, the young man urging her toward a commitment, had she had a serious boyfriend. He had been patient with her need to proceed slowly, but, since they had dated several years, he felt justified in asking her to make a decision about him. Faced with this decision, her symptoms flared with new intensity.

The clinical work got off to a shaky start. The level of Ms. J.'s anxiety was such that talking was almost impossible; tension in her throat made it difficult to vocalize or swallow. Talk of her impending engagement exacerbated her colitis, causing her to have to leave the session to go to the bathroom. During long silences, in which she stared intently at the social worker as if trying to take her in, the worker reassured Ms. J. that they would take their time getting to know each other.

A few weeks into treatment, Ms. J. brought in a poem expressing her defensive need to close herself off from the worker:

I opened the door ever so slightly and saw you
Standing there.
Smiling, you did not stir,
Only your hand moved imperceptibly toward me.
Then you waited patiently.
Fearful of the hand that slaps, I turned away.
The door between us closed quietly.

When the worker thanked her for sharing the poem, Ms. J. was obviously surprised. She expressed a fear that the worker would laugh at her and criticize her feelings. Beginning to cry, she revealed that bringing in the poem came only after a painful struggle. She imagined that the worker would not take the time to read the poem and, if she did, that she would criticize her vulnerable feelings. The worker asked why she felt she had to close the door to others in order to find herself, as described in the poem. She replied that she was afraid to let others in and risk that her feelings would be labeled "stupid." She remembered her mother's typical response to her attempts to tell her how she was feeling: "That's a ridiculous way to feel!" She sobbed as she recalled being yelled at for crying as a little child and sometimes being sent out of the room until she had regained control.

As she talked about fears of being "slapped" by the social worker, Ms. J. began to be more open with her angry feelings toward her family. With the emergence of these feelings came increasing anxiety between sessions. This anxiety found expression in difficulty falling asleep and a recrudescence of colitis. She struggled to remember the content of each session in order to retain "the feeling of comfort I had when I left you last week." A relaxation tape recorded by the worker helped Ms. J. fall asleep at night and enabled her to recall sessions. With this transitional object for self-soothing, she experienced more continuity between sessions and her anxiety abated.

At the end of eight weeks, Ms. J. was able to accompany Mark to select an engagement ring and to set a wedding date. In the transference, she began to test the worker's reactions to independent strivings. She began to arrive for appointments a few minutes late. In the absence of the worker's comments about this behavior, she announced her lateness with a note of defiance. Occasionally she declared her intention to leave an appointment early. The worker's response was one of equanimity, suggesting that these were Ms. J.'s decisions.

Ms. J. began to feel "resentful that I have to come every week." She began a number of sessions with angry complaints about how difficult it had been for her to get to the appointment. The worker listened sympathetically and wondered aloud if these resentful feelings made her think of anything. She recalled having to become furious and then detached before she could assert herself with her parents. She also recalled, tearfully, how her father used to intercede with her mother on Ms. J.'s behalf, telling her to "lay off" and be more reasonable. When she was about 6 years old, however, her father took Ms. J. aside to tell her he could no longer help in this way: "It's causing too much trouble." She reported feeling "devastated and abandoned, like I'd lost everything." Apparently deciding to "shape up" at the expense of interpersonal closeness, she vowed to herself that she would leave home, live alone, and would neither marry nor have children.

Ms. J. and the worker were able to reconstruct that it was soon after the father's "abandonment" that her fears of death and difficulty going to sleep became pronounced. She recalled feeling a nameless dread—"sort of like I was dead inside." Together, the worker and Ms. J. came to understand that she had misunderstood her father's statement to mean that he no longer loved her. To protect herself against this "death" of his love she resolved never again to become vulnerable through loving; but this defensive dread of the dependence involved in loving left her feeling lifeless and empty inside. Her initial fear of death and of going crazy represented memories of a psychic breakdown that had already occurred. Not until she and the worker could understand that the terror stirred by her love for Mark was illusory and belonged to the past could she begin to consider the realistic possibilities offerred by this relationship in the present.

At the end of his paper on object usage, Winnicott (1971e) concluded that the parents' (and the clinician's) capacity to survive aggression in the relationship without retaliating "places the object outside the area of objects set up by the subject's projective mental mechanisms. In this way a world of shared reality is created which the subject can use" (p. 94). This sequence appears to have unfolded in the relationship between Ms. J. and her social worker. The worker's consistent tolerance for Ms. J.'s regressive periods, including those in which she tested the worker's durability and commitment, enabled Ms. J. to use her as an object for positive identification in a way that she had stopped using previous objects in her life. Having "tested" the worker and finding her to be a separate, self-regulating other unlike earlier caregivers, she could more freely gain access to previously denied and projected angry impulses.

THE ANTISOCIAL TENDENCY

Antisocial behavior is another issue that can be conceptualized as an aspect of object relating and object usage. As detailed in Chapter 3, Winnicott believed that those who lie, steal, or commit destructive acts are unconsciously reasserting a rightful claim to a once available holding environment that has been lost. By acting out in a way that compels others to notice and set firmer limits, the antisocial person is, paradoxically, expressing a kind of hope. The hope embedded in the antisocial act is that the person can reclaim a connection with others who will make it safe to experience and express a range of feelings and impulses. Winnicott (1963c) noted that "acting-out is the alternative to despair" (p. 209). The task for clinicians, therefore, is to provide the opportunity for the client to "reach back to the period before the moment of deprivation and rediscover the good object and the good human controlling environment which by existing originally enabled him or her to experience impulses, including destructive ones" (Winnicott 1984, pp. 110–111). To make this process possible, the clinician must understand and accept the legitimacy of the client's claim to love and reliability from valued objects and must be prepared to offer "an ego-supportive structure that is relatively indestructible" (Winnicott 1963c, p. 208).

With many children who act out in the way Winnicott described, the intervention occurs quite naturally: "In the vast majority of cases the parents or the family or guardians of the child recognize the fact of the 'let-down' (so often unavoidable) and by a period of special management, spoiling, or what could be called mental nursing, they see the child through to a recovery from the trauma" (Winnicott 1963c, p. 207). Frequently, clinical intervention can make use of this natural tendency in caregivers to intervene without specific psychotherapy for the child.

Mr. and Mrs. L., the adoptive parents of 6-year-old Mia, came to a family agency for help with handling their daughter's stealing. Mia had been adopted two years previously when her 19-year-old biological mother had married and returned to her country of origin. She put Mia up for adoption because her new husband could not accept the child's biracial heritage. At first Mia had been a model child: polite, compliant, always smiling, and working hard at her school work. Her parents soon began to feel uncomfortable: "She didn't seem real to us. She was more like a little robot. We would hug her and kiss her and she would be so stiff. She did everything she was supposed to do but there were no feelings. We just hoped that she would thaw out after a while."

After Mia had been with them for eighteen months, Mr. and Mrs. L. began to notice small sums of money missing. Eventually they suspected and confronted Mia, who vehemently denied any wrongdoing. Following a stern but supportive talk with her about the impropriety of stealing, they began to give her a weekly allowance. To their surprise and dismay, not only did the stealing continue but a call from Mia's teacher revealed that Mia had been caught stealing her classmates' lunch money on a few occasions. Again, Mia denied stealing even though she had been "caught in the act." She adamantly refused to talk to the school counselor about this behavior.

The social worker noted that Mr. and Mrs. L. were caring and determined to do everything they could to help Mia. She learned that Mia seldom spoke about her biological family or her feelings about having been placed for adoption. It appeared that her stealing was an important communication. Essentially she was asking, "Will you give me away too?" At another level, of course, she was also saying, "My being placed must have had something to do with the way I behaved. I'd better be perfect this time!" As they reflected with the worker on the meaning of Mia's stealing, Mr. and Mrs. L. quickly understood that only because she was feeling safe enough to begin to trust them could she begin to test their commitment to her. Their "survival" of this test, along with some firm limit setting, enabled her to relinquish this form of "communication" and to be more open and direct in expressing her rage and sadness about the loss of her biological family.

In this case, the parents collaborated with the social worker to reframe the meaning of Mia's behavior. This reframing seemed to put curative factors in motion without engaging Mia herself in treatment. In other instances, direct work with the child may be necessary to facilitate the shift from object relating to object use and to understand and redirect the antisocial tendency.

Dave, a 5-year-old boy, was referred to the school social worker by his kindergarten teacher, who was concerned about his hostile-aggressive behavior toward the girls in his class. He hit them, pinched them, and snatched their belongings. His parents described Dave as "wild and uncontrollable" at home as well. Dave's mother felt helpless in the face of his defiant behavior. Often, when efforts at reasoning with him failed, she would resort to yelling, spanking him, and sending him to his room. There, rather than calm down, he would continue to wreak havoc on his furniture, toys, and clothes.

The developmental history revealed that things had gone well until Dave was about 2. "He was the sweetest baby and then when he hit the terrible twos, all hell broke loose!" Detailed exploration of this period suggested that Dave's behavior was fairly typical of a 2-year-old trying to assert his independence, test limits, and explore his expanding world. But when the family moved to a larger house, the father began working longer hours to pay the mortgage, and a baby sister arrived, Dave's assertiveness escalated in intensity to more frequent hostile-aggressive outbursts.

Initially the social worker met with Dave's parents and his

teacher to help them develop a plan for managing Dave's behavior. This plan included providing him ample advance notice to prepare for activities he found difficult, offering him choices rather than telling him what to do, and providing small rewards for successes rather than threatening him with punishment for misbehavior. Episodes of destructive aggression were to be handled by holding Dave and talking to him about his feelings. If too upset to talk, alternatives such as drawing a picture or punching a cushion were to be provided. The goal was to help Dave identify his upsetting affects and, in collaboration with an empathic adult, verbalize or symbolize rather than act them out destructively. The parents were encouraged to sign Dave up for a neighborhood sports league where his aggressive and competitive strivings could be channeled into an activity he and his father could share. The mother was referred to a baby-sitting cooperative that met monthly to discuss parenting issues.

With these supports in place, the social worker began meeting weekly with Dave for play therapy. He was resistant at first, calling the worker "stupid poopy face" and threatening to mobilize his superheroes to wreck her office. He began each session by "accidentally" knocking something off the worker's desk or bumping into her or her furniture. At first the worker was tentative, offering Dave gentle interpretations of his anger. After one particularly trying session Dave yelled, "You're too nice to help me! You let me keep doing stuff—I don't want to come here anymore!" Startled by Dave's appraisal of her, the worker gave careful thought to her feelings about him. She recognized that she didn't feel very "nice." She was, in fact, angered by his constant provocations. She wondered why she had not set firm limits with Dave and realized that she felt guilty about her anger toward him. Her "niceness" was not genuine but rather a reaction formation to her own uncomfortable angry feelings.

This self-awareness enabled the worker to become very clear and tough with Dave about not hurting her or the office. Dave responded by challenging each limit with tremendous energy. The worker periodically doubted her capacity to survive, but, fortified by her understanding that he needed to test her durability, she held her ground in every skirmish. After five weeks of battle, Dave began to talk more. He complained bitterly about his little sister, expressing particular outrage over his perception that, no matter how "bad" she was, she was never punished. He drew pictures of her stealing his toys and breaking up his room. He built an air force of paper planes to protect his property and confided to the social worker that she did not have to worry about her own safety—"I'll protect you, too." In conjunction with these developments, his behavior in school and at home improved dramatically.

Over the next few weeks Dave acknowledged that he gave his mother a hard time and wondered if he should be sent away: "Her life would probably be better if she didn't have me. When she says, 'I just don't know what to do with you,' I feel scared. I jump around a lot to get rid of the butterflies in my tummy. Sometimes I'm just so bad I make Mommy cry; then she gets mad and spanks me." The spankings hurt and made Dave "mad," and, though he seemed to quiet down afterward, he felt lonely and "bad." He confessed that, when his teacher used to send him to the hall to sit by himself, he felt similarly. Now she held him and talked firmly. Dave squirmed around and "once I kicked her. I felt scared I'd hurt her." When she responded by "holding on tight" he felt calmer: "At first the butterflies get worse when she holds me but then they fly away."

By the end of the school year Dave had made progress at controlling his destructive feelings. He wrote a story about going with his teacher on a rocketship to the moon. At home there were still difficult times, and the school social worker met with Dave's parents to recommend continued work at a family service agency over the summer.

This case illustrates Winnicott's hypothesis that children who begin to act out antisocially are responding to the loss of a previously stable holding environment and associated ego relatedness. Dave's world was a reliable place until the family moved, the father began working more, and he lost his primary position with the parents to his new sister. In reaction to this perceived deprivation, Dave's normal assertiveness shifted to destructive aggressiveness, some of it displaced from his envied sister to girls at school—and from his mother to the female teacher. He seemed to be demanding that his environment notice and "hold" him.

The social worker's treatment plan and interventions were informed by her understanding that, in order for Dave to "use" her and others for further development, they had to demonstrate their durability, and, thus, their separateness from his projected "bad" impulses. At first, the worker felt guilty about her own angry feelings toward Dave, thus identifying with his projection of himself as "bad." Later, her insight about the meaning of her guilt and associated passivity enabled her to set appropriate limits and, ultimately, to survive Dave's aggressive attacks without retaliating. Dave's subsequent experience of being safely held by the worker, the teacher, and the parents enabled him to get more of his impulses into symbolic form through language and play and to contain his anxiety—the "butterflies"—until it abated. This containment, in turn, facilitated development of appropriate guilt feelings, wishes to protect others, and a capacity for concern.

The following case depicts elements of the antisocial tendency in an adult client.

> Mr. S., a 30-year-old married man with two children, was referred for social work services by the physician who was treating him for a back injury in a hospital rehabilitation unit. Mr. S. complained of severe back pain that prevented him from sleeping and caused irritability toward his wife and children, a sense of hopelessness about his future, and anger toward his former employer, his lawyer, and his parole officer. His sexual performance was impaired by the injury, and he felt humiliated because his wife was working outside the home while he cared for the children.
>
> Asked to provide a history, Mr. S. described his father as having been physically abusive and alcoholic. He recalled periods during his childhood when he was sent to retrieve him from a local bar two or three times a week. His mother and

grandmother had "great hopes" for Mr. S. and, together, provided a source of stability. Both had helped him financially since he had become unable to work. He noted that, during his growing up, his mother had not been able to set limits on him or his brothers. Mr. S. had used drugs and alcohol to excess since adolescence.

Prior to his back injury Mr. S.'s family life had been chaotic. His wife left him several times after he beat her and he had been incarcerated for two weeks after a repeat offense of drunk driving. At the time of referral he was on parole and his driver's license had been revoked.

In the initial session with the social worker, Mr. S. revealed that he was taking an "occasional drink" and that he was driving to the hospital daily for his rehabilitation therapy. His obvious discomfort in describing this suggested that he was asking for help in controlling his impulsive, self-destructive behavior. Tearfully, he told of his fantasy that God was punishing him for his wicked past. To the worker, this remorse was a hopeful sign, indicating a possible capacity to use treatment. A stated wish to "make it up to my wife and kids for the hell I've put them through" also indicated a wish to make reparation. He feared his wife would leave him and questioned whether the worker would want to make a second appointment "now that you know what sort of character you're dealing with." While his mother had never given up on him, he felt he had "worn her down"— used her up and "destroyed" her as a previously available object. In the sessions, he expressed rage at the mother for allowing his father to abuse her and the children and for letting Mr. S. himself "get away with murder."

Feeling acutely upset in one session, he began banging his fist on the worker's desk and expressed an urge to go out and get "stinking drunk" so he wouldn't care any more. He did, however, respond to the worker's calm observation that when he felt anxious he became angry and sought to numb the intensity of his feelings with alcohol. She stressed the importance of talking about rather than acting on these feelings. She indicated she could not sanction his driving to appointments without a license and after drinking, thus setting limits in a way the mother and grandmother had been unable to. These interventions had the effect of defusing his anger, and he became more thoughtful. Ultimately they explored the meaning of Mr. S.'s antisocial behavior. Through spouse abuse, drinking, and driving without a license, Mr. S. seemed to be communicating a demand that society catch and "hold" him, as he hoped his parents would. Through antisocial behavior, he continued to express that hope, but in a way that was destructive to others. Since a lack of earlier limits had compromised superego development, he relied on external controls to help him contain and manage anxiety aroused by strong affects. Unfortunately, gaps in the legal system made it possible for him to continue this maladaptive pattern in ways that fostered rather than limited his acting on poorly integrated impulses. Fortunately, he was able to use the relationship with the worker to begin to reflect rather than act upon his feelings.

BROADER APPLICATIONS

In addressing the antisocial tendency in human behavior, individual treatment should be augmented by intervention at the community/society level. Such intervention must be informed by a developmental perspective on the *meaning* of antisocial acting-out. Winnicott (1963c) emphasized that the seed of antisocial behavior is suffering—the pain, depression, and rage associated with the person's "correct perception at a time in early childhood that at first all was well, or well enough, and then that all was not well" (p. 207). He also spoke of the antisocial individual's "need to make society acknowledge and repay" (p. 207). Unfortunately, a too-frequent response to this need is retaliation rather than understanding. This can take the form of revenge and punishment or, more subtly, a determination to resocialize people without acknowledging the original trauma or deprivation.

Winnicott's formulation allows us to place the antisocial tendency, then, not in the individual but in the intermediate area between the individual and society. As a consequence, treatment that addresses only the individual's difficulties remains incomplete. To generate a capacity for concern in individuals requires expressions of concern by society. Individual and family interventions, therefore, must be augmented by policy initiatives that humanize the legal and criminal justice systems.

In conclusion, it is important to note that in human development the move from object relating to object use is never complete. Important others, inevitably, are always in part subjectively conceived. Others are perceived and interpreted on the basis of the individual's unique experiences with them and the resulting projections and projective identifications. This phenomenon occurs not just at the individual level but, as suggested by Ross (in press), Volkan (1988), and other scholars applying psychodynamic theory to sociocultural conflict, at the level of national and international relations. Here, deprivation or trauma imposed on one social, ethnic, religious, or national group by another can set off mutually destructive aggression that can fuel enmity, if not war, for generations.

For societies as well as individuals, the capacity to view others more objectively, to acknowledge them as self-regulating, separate entities, and to develop empathy and concern for them is a developmental achievement that offers another level of depth and complexity to relationships. But this objectivity is invariably tinged with subjective distortion. Most relationships are comprised of a rich mix of subjective and objective perceptions. The move from object relating to object use, if successfully navigated and internalized, makes possible the existence of a dynamic potential space in relationships at all levels—a space wherein, a degree of expectable but negotiable conflict notwithstanding, personal and interpersonal authenticity and relative harmony can predominate.

8

THE TRUE AND FALSE SELF

In Marjorie Williams's (1975) well-known children's book, *The Velveteen Rabbit*, we find the following exchange about becoming real:

"What is real?" asked the Rabbit one day . . . "Does it mean having things that buzz inside you and a stick-out handle?"

"Real isn't how you are made," said the Skin Horse. "It's a thing that happens to you. When a child loves you for a long, long time, not just to play with, but *really* loves you, then you become real."

"Does it hurt?" asked the Rabbit.

"Sometimes," said the Skin Horse, for he was always truthful. "When you are real you don't mind being hurt."

"Does it happen all at once, like being wound up," he asked, "or bit by bit?"

"It doesn't happen all at once," said the Skin Horse. "You become. It takes a long time . . . . but once you are real you can't become unreal again. It lasts for always" (pp. 17–20).

Winnicott (1971a) wrote that "feeling real is more than existing; it is finding a way to exist as oneself, and to relate to objects as oneself, and to have a self into which to retreat for relaxation" (p. 117). As he saw it, the developmental basis for feeling real is the true self. With this concept, implied in all of his work but developed most thoroughly late in his career, Winnicott tackled an issue that has preoccupied philosophers for centuries. Characteristically, he put his own stamp on it. He attempted to describe how the self, at birth only an inchoate potential, finds full realization in a world of shared reality. At first, "the True Self comes from the aliveness of the body tissues and the working of body-functions, including the heart's action and breathing" (Winnicott 1960b, p. 148). Then, as described in previous chapters, this sensorimotor and sensoritonic aliveness finds increased definition through the process of being gathered together by the caregiver's sensitive holding, handling, and object presenting. A crucial aspect of these activities is the visual and kinesthetic mirroring that accompanies them, a process through which the infant discovers his or her emotional life in the caregiver's eyes, facial expressions, and attuned ministrations.

Mahler viewed this multimodal mirroring as a vital aspect of psychic development during the symbiotic phase, when the infant periodically experiences affirmation of a dual unity with the caregiver by "seeing" him- or herself as a gleam in her eye (see Wolman 1991). Kohut (1971, 1977) also emphasized the importance of mirroring as essential to the development of a cohesive self. He believed that insufficient early mirroring sets the stage for a lifelong susceptibility to fragmentation in psychologically stressful situations. When mirroring is successful, the baby learns to integrate somatic and psychological phenomena. As Sacksteder (1989) puts it, "A mother with her baby is constantly introducing and reintroducing the baby's body and psyche to each other" (p. 371).

As she receives, reflects, and celebrates her infant's spontaneous gestures and thus cultivates an illusion of omnipotence, the caregiver fosters an ego relatedness that strengthens his or her capacity to be alone in the intimate presence of another. Then, as she gradually de-adapts to this illusion and accepts and supports his or her attachments to substitute objects, she facilitates the development of a transitional process. This process gives birth to a capacity for symbolization, self-soothing, and, with internalization and resulting intrapsychic structure, the eventual capacity to be alone comfortably either in the presence or absence of others.

Finally, the true self is consolidated through the caregiver's non-retaliatory survival of the baby's normal aggression and associated destructive testing of her durability. With the caregiver's survival, the baby begins to experience empathy and concern for others as individuals with an internal life of their own. Through thus rendering the other more objective, more "real," the reality of the self is further affirmed. And, as Winnicott (1960b) suggested, "Every new period of living in which the True Self has not been seriously interrupted results in a strengthening of the sense of being real" (p. 149).

The outcome of serious interruptions of the true self, Winnicott believed, is the development of a false self identity. He made clear that, depending on the stage at which interruptions occur, there are degrees of false self development. These range from states in which the individual's entire identity is falsely grounded to the mutually acknowledged and accepted falsity that characterizes civilized social interaction. The clinical material that follows is organized according to these levels of false self development.

THE TRUE SELF IN COMPLETE DISGUISE

When there is interruption or impingement in earliest development—when, for example, the caregiver fails to notice and affirm the infant's spontaneous gestures and, instead, repeatedly substitutes her own gestures to which the infant must react—there may develop "the truly split-off compliant False Self which is taken for the whole child" (Winnicott 1960b, p. 150). With ego relatedness compromised in this manner, spontaneity is foreclosed, the true self is hidden, and "extreme restlessness, an inability to concentrate, and a need to collect impingements from external reality so that living-time of the individual can be filled by reactions to these impingements" results (Winnicott 1960b, p. 150). In adult clients presenting this configuration, behavior and experience seem not to emanate from within, but rather in reaction to external demands or conventions. These are the so-called "as-if" personalities, perhaps socially competent and occupationally successful, but lacking a sense of personal solidity and aliveness. In the countertransference, such clients may evoke feelings of detachment, an eerie sense that one is alone in the room, or inordinate difficulty coming up with a preliminary formulation of core issues and dynamics.

Mrs. B., a 60-year-old woman, came to a church-affiliated counseling service a few months after her husband left her, declaring that he "couldn't take it any more." Although they had been married thirty-five years, Mrs. B. had no idea that there were problems. Her husband was a busy physician who worked long hours until his semi-retirement a few months prior to the first appointment. Mrs. B. had devoted her life to her four children, now grown and married, and to her husband's career. She entertained business associates, helped in the office, edited his professional papers, and accompanied him to conferences. When asked to describe how she experienced their relationship, she appeared puzzled: "We were just like any other couple. What is it you want to know?" She reported few interests of her own and now felt lost.

As she told her story, Mrs. B. shifted around in her chair, her eyes darting restlessly from the social worker to various objects in the office that she would ask about. She interrupted herself to ask the worker what he did about his paper work and whether or not he had a wife to help. When he tried to elicit further information from her, Mrs. B. interrupted him with obvious annoyance. At the end of the first session the worker felt somewhat dazed and at a loss to focus on Mrs. B.'s core issues. He had a sense of the kinds of activities with which she filled her life, but he knew nothing of her inner life. When asked questions such as what was that like for you, or how did you feel when that happened, she became indignant and retorted, "How do you think I felt!" or "How would you feel if someone did that to you?" She appeared to feel attacked by the worker's attempts to get to know her and her defensive response was to counterattack. At one point she said, "Look, I don't want you to waste my time asking a lot of silly questions. I just want you to tell me what I need to do to get my life back to normal."

To the worker it seemed that when Mrs. B.'s husband left he took with him his wife's sense of identity. By building her life around his professional persona, she had found a context in which to sustain a false self. Without him, she felt adrift. With the social worker, she seemed unable to voice her own experience and, thus, made a dynamic formulation of her situation very difficult.

THE FALSE SELF IN ANOREXIA NERVOSA

The most serious level of false self identity disturbance, that in which the false self is all that is experienced by the person and seen by others, may appear in cases where there has been a failure of personalization and a consequent dissociation between psyche and soma. The true self is, first of all, a body-self. That we locate a sense of self in the body is one of those day-to-day phenomena that most people take for granted. But for people whose early development has been characterized by an environment wherein caregivers have not received and responded to the spontaneous gestures of the body-based true self, psyche and soma may be split off from each other. As Sacksteder (1989) suggests, for these people the sense of self or personality is not experienced as localized in the body. He believes this psychosomatic estrangement to characterize some clients with anorexia nervosa. Rather than feeling grounded in and positive toward the body as an extension of self, they view the body as an enemy—"as a source of embarrassment, shame, anxiety, humiliation, pain, or ruin" (p. 367). The effort to starve this enemy of the psyche represents in these individuals an effort to control and dominate a fearsome, alien force. For Janette, described below, achieving a normal weight appeared to represent the betrayal of a pact with her mother—a pact to remain a narcissistic extension of the mother rather than develop into a person in her own right.

At the time of her admission to a psychiatric hospital, Janette, age 18, was 5 feet 9 inches tall but weighed only 82 pounds. She had the pallor and tell-tale skeletal appearance of severe anorexia, and there were multiple ulcerations on her arms and legs where her skin had begun to break down. In jarring contrast with this deterioration were her perfect clothing, makeup, and grooming. Her expensive suit and matching accessories, in conjunction with an oddly affectless, mechanical presentation, gave her the appearance of an emaciated mannequin.

The social worker and psychiatrist who greeted Janette and her parents were struck by the remarkable resemblance between her and her mother. Though the mother was at a normal weight, in other respects they were nearly identical. In addition to similar expensive clothing, both wore makeup more suitable to evening wear than to a hospital admission. The two sat together, exchanging knowing smiles, while the father appeared disconnected and depressed. It soon became clear that it was the father, at the urging of the family physician, who was pressing for hospitalization. Janette seemed puzzled about all the fuss over her "thinness." And her mother, though claiming to realize the seriousness of Janette's condition, quipped cheerfully to the admissions team, "You can't be too rich or too thin!"

Both mother and daughter were tearful when the time came for Janette to go to her hospital room and for the parents to meet separately with the social worker before returning to their home in another state. Janette was assured by her mother, "You'll be out of here in no time; all you need is a little rest and a few good meals!" After Janette went up to her room, her mother was inconsolable—"I can't imagine a day without her!"

In subsequent appointments with the parents, the social worker learned that, as an only child, Janette was her mother's "best friend." They shopped together daily, acquiring clothes and makeup, and were referred to as twins by people at the beauty parlor they frequented. Neither had close friends outside this dyad. While the parents claimed to have a good marriage, it appeared to succeed only due to the father's tacit agreement not to intrude on the mother–daughter relationship and his willingness to support their lavish lifestyle by putting in long hours at his company.

In the hospital, Janette remained isolated, depressed, and homesick. She stayed at the periphery of activities and kept her distance from the staff. In meetings, staff members reported frustration at their inability to make contact with Janette. They described her as mechanical and doll-like, a "perfect," benignly pleasant, but unapproachable presence on the unit. Any time during the day that she was not in scheduled activities, she retreated to her room to work on her makeup and nails.

Meanwhile, the social worker was faced with the management of the parents' resistance to the treatment plan, which included regulation of the frequency and duration of visits with Janette. The mother could not understand the need for planned separation, and the father could not challenge the mother's demands to see Janette more frequently. As a way to sustain connection, the mother sent daily care packages of makeup kits, clothes, jewelry, and other accessories. She was incredulous and angry when these were intercepted by nursing staff and returned. Efforts to help the mother understand that staff were trying to help Janette look beneath her polished exterior at some of her feelings and issues were met with denial—"there's no harm in making sure she looks as pretty as possible!" Occasionally Janette's mother would appear unannounced to surprise her daughter, then would be devastated to find her away at an off-site activity or otherwise unavailable.

With the enforced hiatus in their nearly symbiotic relationship, Janette's mother became increasingly depressed. Since she refused referral for psychotherapy, the hospital social worker began to see her individually during visits. In these sessions she revealed an early life of deprivation and unhappiness. As a young woman she had fled her family and pursued a modeling career. She became obsessed by her appearance and, although never anorexic, was preoccupied by her weight. In the early years of her marriage she became pregnant seven times and, worried about the impact on her appearance and career, ended each pregnancy through abortion. She spoke of these abortions in a detached way, apparently ascribing little meaning to them.

When Janette's mother stopped working and "the time was right," the couple decided to have a child. They hoped for a daughter and were ecstatic with Janette's birth. She was viewed, especially by the mother, as a "perfect doll" who must be kept clean, quiet, and beautifully adorned. It was distressing for the mother, therefore, when Janette began to experience eating difficulties as an infant. She would frequently spit up her food and was fussy. Although some eating problems persisted through toddlerhood, they abated by the time Janette entered school. A picture of 6-year-old Janette standing by her school bus revealed an oddly stilted, unsmiling, but perfectly turned-out "doll." Things seemed to go well enough during grade school, although teachers repeatedly sent home reports that Janette was not working up to her potential. It was at puberty that problems again began to surface visibly. Menarche was extremely upsetting to Janette, and as her body began to develop she became more and more isolated from peers at school. She lost weight, but stayed within normal limits until six months before the admission, when, at about the time she began to explore going away to college, she started to diet and exercise compulsively. She experienced dramatic weight loss, her menses ceased, and she became increasingly phobic about leaving home.

The hospital staff's efforts to help Janette gain weight and understand herself, as well as efforts to help the parents separate enough to permit her to engage fully in treatment, were unsuccessful. Although she gained some weight and went through the motions of hospital activities, she remained detached and deanimated. Despite the social worker's efforts to assist the parents in helping her remain, Janette left the hospital against medical advice.

Janette, rather than realizing a true self of her own, appeared to have evolved a false self consistent with her mother's demands for a "perfect doll." We can hypothesize that the mother was unable to recognize and support spontaneous gestures that did not confirm her image of her infant as doll-like. Janette's early feeding difficulties suggest possible disturbances in the mother–infant relationship. Spitting up may have been a sort of spontaneous gesture, an early expression of assertion or failure to comply with the mother's rigidity. It is unlikely that her mother coped comfortably with this behavior, given the value she placed on docility, cleanliness, and perfection of appearance. More likely, she foreclosed Janette's true self expressions, substituting her own demands for a "doll" who would mirror her own composure and beauty.

The mother's descriptions of her aborted pregnancies suggested that she did not view them as "real"; similarly, she did not seem to view Janette as a "real" human being with an inner life and developmental agenda of her own. Janette was to be the mother's companion, recruited as a narcissistic extension. This contract appeared to work well enough until Janette's puberty, when she began visibly to develop. It was as though her body turned on her, urging her to break the compact with her mother to remain her "perfect doll." Failing to make use of the "second individuation" of adolescence to achieve a degree of separation (Blos 1967), Janette became even more enmeshed with her mother. The father's collusion in supporting their symbiosis reflected his own more successfully concealed separation difficulties. Janette seemed to be trying to control and shrink her body, reflecting a cognitive regression to a concrete perception of her body as distinct from her self. The extent of this dissociation and resulting distorted perception was revealed in her denial of the drastic changes in her appearance.

The separation enforced by Janette's hospitalization catalyzed depression both in her and in her mother, whose intrusiveness mitigated against staff efforts to help Janette have her own treatment experience. Good at complying, she went along with prescribed routines, but there appeared to be no real or true self to engage. And, as Horner (1979) notes, "until one can make contact with the real self, there is no treatment" (p. 206). In retrospect, this family might have benefited from an approach wherein all three could have been hospitalized and separation-individuation and the resistances to it could have been addressed in more tolerable increments.

THE FALSE SELF AS PROTECTOR OF THE TRUE SELF

Less extreme is a false self whose role is to protect and defend the true self. Here the true self is not closed off from awareness but is acknowledged by the person and allowed a secret life. A person with this configuration presents a false self to the world in order to prevent detection of fragile true self aspects and to protect the true self from a potentially harmful environment. The person is aware, however, of who the true self is. Clinically, the presentation may be guarded, even aloof, but beneath this may exist a sense of vulnerability, accessibility, and a potential for engagement.

In some instances, only confrontation can penetrate a false self presentation. In the instance described below, the client kept the social worker at a distance and managed her own feelings of helplessness and vulnerability through aloofness.

Ms. N., a 52-year-old divorcee, came to a suburban family
service agency for help in smoothing the post-divorce adjustment for herself and her two children, a son, 11, and a daughter, 15. Ms. N.'s presentation was one of reserve and cool control. She was unfailingly polite, but there was an icy veneer to
her manner that made her feel unapproachable to the young
male social worker assigned to her. Although she rarely missed
an appointment, she seemed detached. She was impeccably
dressed and groomed despite living on only a small salary from
her job as a sales clerk and minimal child support. The worker
thought of her as his "perfect" client.

Ms. N. harbored considerable hostility for her ex-husband
and spent much of each session in vitriolic disparagement of
him and, as she put it, of "most other men." The worker's efforts
to direct her attention to the hurt and loneliness she felt were
dismissed as irrelevant. "You can't possibly know or understand
what I feel." The worker found it difficult to sustain empathy
in the face of her seeming disregard. He began to think of her
as arrogant and narcissistic and became aware of dreading their
sessions. It did not occur to him to address her presentation as
an issue in their relationship or to consider it as a form of communication about the way she may have been treated in other
relationships. Instead he mused to himself that he could well
understand why her husband left her.

After several months of treatment, Ms. N.'s daughter began to
act out in school. The school counselor called Ms. N. in and suggested that she get help for her. Ms. N. then asked the social worker
to recommend someone on the agency staff. Surprised and gratified by this rare vote of confidence in him, the worker gave much
thought to this referral and made painstaking efforts to arrange
a good match. He spoke at length with the prospective clinician,
a capable 27-year-old female social worker who had worked in
school settings, and made sure she had a full history and other
relevant information. He intended this to be a "perfect" referral.

Predictably, things did not go well. Ms. N. was livid when she
came for her next appointment a few days after her daughter's
first visit. Having been in the waiting room when the new worker
came to meet her daughter, Ms. N. was surprised and disappointed: "I couldn't believe who you picked for her! She's so

young, so bright-eyed, so obviously inexperienced—she couldn't possibly help Tammy! They're practically the same age!" The worker, in shock, tried to listen quietly. His absence of response seemed to inflame Ms. N. further: "Then Tammy told me that this 'therapist' said that kids sometimes need to bend the rules. That did it for me! You really blew it; my one chance to get help for my daughter and you pick this inept youngster!"

The worker felt, first, unjustifiably attacked, then wounded, then furious. Overcome by a surge of anger, his voice was shaking when he finally spoke: "Your reaction to this is way out of line! I don't know why you would make such accusations about my colleague and about me. You do all you can to keep me at a distance. After all these months it's as though we have no relationship at all. I have a strong feeling you'd have found fault with anyone I selected. Your attitude is very hard to take!"

The worker was startled by this uncharacteristic outburst and immediately experienced intense remorse at his loss of control. He felt he'd violated all his standards of professional conduct. Worse, he believed he had retaliated against rather than survived Ms. N.'s attack on his competence. He had reacted rather than reflected. To his surprise Ms. N., although obviously shaken, did not stride out of the office. She seemed thoughtful for a moment, then asked a few questions about the daughter's worker's qualifications and experience. Finally, she said, "Tammy is so different from me—always testing the rules, talking back, showing her colors. I just don't know how to handle her and would love someone to do it for me." The worker experienced, for the first time, an infusion of empathy for Ms. N.'s isolation and her struggles as a single parent. His confrontation had broken a barrier between them. In subsequent interviews Ms. N. talked more openly about her feelings of regret about her divorce, her worries about her children and her aging parents, and fears of starting over in mid-life.

In this case, the worker's confrontation served to penetrate a false-self facade that Ms. N. had erected to protect herself from a range of painful feelings. Although Ms. N.'s style remained one of relative formality, she felt more real to the worker. The intervention, though unplanned and potentially hurtful, created the potential therapeutic space for authentic exchange. Gradually it became clear that by setting up conditions in which the worker felt dismissed, irrelevant, and invalidated, Ms. N. was letting him know how she felt when her husband left her for a much younger woman. The worker further realized that Ms. N. projected her own feelings of ineptitude onto her daughter's worker—a young, enthusiastic woman who might further humiliate and supersede her, as did her husband's paramour. In contrast to the previous case, this client had developed a differentiated sense of self, but she had developed a distancing facade as a way of protecting it from exposure and potential harm.

The social worker was fortunate that his unplanned intervention led to a good result. Indeed, it had a quality of retaliation. Ideally, the kind of strain emerging in the therapeutic relationship should have been taken up reflectively at an earlier point—perhaps around Ms. N.'s disparaging references to "all men," which, at some level, undoubtedly included the worker. This is another instance in which consultation and supervision can be invaluable in helping clinicians monitor and manage their own countertransference issues.

THE FALSE SELF IN SEARCH OF THE TRUE SELF

In the segment of the continuum called "more toward health," Winnicott (1960b, p. 143) hypothesized a false self whose main concern is to search out conditions that will make it possible for the true self to find expression. The person employs compliant or acquiescent behaviors, in other words, not to survive or protect a secret self, but to pave the way for true self expression. Winnicott (1960b) believed that when these efforts fail and people cannot protect the true self from exploitation, they may turn to a kind of redemptive suicide: "Suicide in this context is the destruction of the total self in avoidance of annihilation of the True Self" (p. 143).

Mr. K. came to an emergency service asking to be hospitalized because he feared that he would kill himself. He had become despondent and suicidal after the woman he had been dating for several months told him that she thought he was a wonderful person but that she needed someone who thought for himself and was more spontaneous. Mr. K. felt devastated—his sense of the relationship was that he had finally found someone with whom he could feel safe enough to "be himself." He had begun taking small risks, such as ordering what he wanted from a restaurant menu rather than checking with his date to learn what she'd prefer and what she might want to sample from his plate. He understood her criticism but could not believe that she had no faith that he could change. When she said, "Who you are is not what I want," he felt like his core self had been annihilated: "It was as though a knife had been plunged into my heart."

Now he was obsessed by the fantasy of turning a knife on himself, a preoccupation that had its antecedent in a childhood incident. He recalled that as a child of 8 he had stood in the kitchen, a knife poised in his hand and pointed at his chest. This incident followed his mother's declaration, after he had done something that angered her, that "I don't know you; get out of my sight!" As much as it expressed compliance with his mother's wish that he disappear, Mr. K.'s suicidal gesture seemed to be a way to preserve himself in a way over which he had ultimate control.

More routinely in outpatient settings of all kinds, social workers see clients whose true self has developed to an extent but who learned early to disguise it from detection for fear of reactivating feelings associated with earlier trauma. Such clients often maintain postures of tireless compliance to others' demands. As one worn-out mother and career woman put it, "I never even think about saying no. If I did, people might not like me. I'd be left all alone with no family and no friends." Exploration of her fears of abandonment revealed that her parents had died when she was 9 years old and that she, along with her younger siblings, had been placed in foster care. Despite a cognitive awareness that the parents died from an infectious illness that she could not have prevented, she continued to feel partly responsible. "I didn't help them out enough in the store. They got worn out and died. If only I had done more they might have lived longer." In adult life she was driven to conceal her "true"— as she saw it, irresponsible and neglectful—nature from herself and others as a way to manage her guilt.

Also seen frequently are clients who, although it is apparent to the clinician that there is a nascent true self, feel as though at bottom they are empty and fraudulent. They frantically try to assess the wishes of others so that they can comply and experience acute distress if clues as to how they should behave are not apparent.

> Ms. Y., 27, sought counseling because of immobilizing anxiety in her job as a teacher's assistant. She worried endlessly about her supervisor's opinion of her: "I sit in staff meetings studying her face so that I can figure out what she wants from me. I'm afraid if I speak up with my own ideas everyone will shout me down." Although intelligent and capable, she had been unable to finish college due to her difficulty completing assignments. Sitting down to write, she began anticipating her professor's potential criticisms and tried to make her work fit what she imagined to be perfectionistic expectations. "The more freedom I was given with an assignment the worse it was. I looked into myself for ideas and found nothing!"
>
> As the social worker explored Ms. Y.'s sense of inauthenticity and lack of confidence, she learned that "the only person I can remember being myself with is my dad, but he died when I was 6. We had a lot of fun just being silly with each other. I'd make things up and he'd go along with it. You know, just enter into the spirit of being a kid with me. After my dad died and there

was just my mother and me, I was always having to figure out what she was feeling and then how to act. I could tell when she was getting angry and I'd say things to try and calm her down. Sometimes I'd get so mad at her I'd say to myself, 'What about me? Aren't I a person too?' Then I'd ask her for something I wanted and she'd throw a fit. I'd end up saying, 'It's okay, I didn't really mean it.'"

To preserve her ties with her grieving, self-absorbed mother, Ms. Y. learned to suppress her own needs. The mother's emotional state was so fragile following her husband's death that she subsumed her daughter's needs to her own. Ms. Y. recalled going on a nature walk with her mother: "She wouldn't let me stop to go to the bathroom until she needed to go." Even her ideas, if different from her mother's, elicited impatience; so she learned to keep them to herself.

This defensive denial of her own thoughts and feelings appeared early in the transference. Repeatedly, Ms. Y. asked the social worker how she thought particular situations should be handled: "Do you think I should have said something? Was I wrong in thinking that?" The worker felt pressured, almost coerced, and at times quite irritated. Reflecting on these reactions, she realized that she was feeling intense anxiety reactive to the desperation beneath Ms. Y.'s insistence on being told what to do. When the worker responded, "Your questions are important, but I think we need to understand why you so urgently need me to provide the answers," Ms. Y. seemed immobilized. "I feel like you're leaving me in a black, empty void." On the other hand she recalled that when a previous therapist had given her answers and advice, "that didn't feel so good either. It was like I didn't exist unless he gave me permission."

Here, the social worker's task was to provide a safe and supportive, but nondirective context in which Ms. Y. could begin to risk expressing her own thoughts and feelings. The worker's abstention from giving her advice and suggestions was at first experienced as depriving and frightening. Yet Ms. Y. recognized at some level that receiving such guidance would continue to impede her development as a person in her own right. Ms. Y. had learned to live a reactive rather than a creative life. That she could remember the capacity to engage in spontaneous, playful interactions with her father suggested to the worker that a true self existed but had been suppressed. The worker's invitation for Ms. Y. to reflect on her need for someone to tell her what to do was an invitation to begin to play, again, with her ideas and impulses.

> A pattern began to emerge wherein Ms. Y. would come in, talk spontaneously for several minutes, and then become distressed by the worker's silence. "Why am I doing all the talking? It bothers me when you're quiet and I don't know what you're thinking." When the worker responded that she thought it important not to interrupt Ms. Y. but to give her the opportunity to talk for as long as she needed to express her ideas, there was a silence followed by, "But I end up feeling that I've lost you and worrying that you're sitting there getting bored or even mad with me!" It took several sessions for her to integrate the new experience of being truly listened to. Soon, however, she began to tell humorous anecdotes. She seemed amazed when the worker laughed, and needed to make sure that this kind of play was acceptable. "Are we allowed to do this? Are you sure I'm not wasting your time?"

THE CARETAKER SELF

Another frequent clinical manifestation of the false self at this level is the caretaker adaptation. This may find expression not only in the client's external life but in the therapeutic relationship as well. Here, the client may be looking to treatment as a place where the true self can find realization, but a lifelong defense of tending to others as a way of disguising and protecting the true self gets in the way. As children, these clients have developed a pseudomaturity that leads to praise for their self-sufficiency and precocity. In the clinical relationship as adults, they present themselves as easy or "good" clients—verbal, reflective, cooperative, undemanding—who can deflect clinicians from probing for and exploring real issues. This presentation often replicates an earlier object relationship based on the client's having been a caretaker to his or her parents in childhood. In the transference, the client "takes care" of the clinician, thus demonstrating what went on in earlier significant relationships. In the countertransference, the clinician may permit him- or herself to be taken care of in this manner, acting out the earlier dynamic and being deterred from the work of addressing key, true self issues.

Ms. H., a 25-year-old secretary, came to a family agency after being laid off from her job. Although her employer explained to her that her dismissal was related to cutbacks and her lack of longevity at the job, Ms. H. felt devastated: "I just don't understand—I did everything right, was always on time, stayed late when they needed me, worked for others when they wanted a day off. . . . I guess it just wasn't enough." She experienced acute anxiety, sleeplessness, and loss of appetite.

The crisis passed quickly; the company's outplacement office helped Ms. H. find a new job. Ms. H. decided to continue seeing the social worker, however, realizing that her reaction had been extreme. Exploration of her history revealed that she had been raised by an aunt and uncle; both parents had died in an automobile accident when she was 2½ years old. Family stories portrayed Ms. H. as an "angel" who "never caused any trouble" and whose self-sufficiency was laudable. The aunt was asthmatic, and Ms. H. quickly assumed the role of looking after her. One of the most frequently told tales of her competence related to a time when, at age 4, Ms. H. called the ambulance and rode with her aunt to the hospital during a particularly severe asthma attack. She described this and similar episodes without reference to any of her own feelings.

As a client, Ms. H. seemed to know from the outset what was expected of her. She was prompt, never cancelled or requested to change an appointment, and invariably paid her fee at the end of each session. She talked at length about her life, her thoughts, and after watching a TV talk show about the meaning of dreams, began to present dreams for "analysis." The social worker's experience was to look forward to his sessions with Ms. H. It was an easy hour, a rarity in his caseload of crisis-ridden families. He eagerly took the dreams to his supervisor, who, although supportive of exploring their meaning, also noted that the work seemed to have no "meat," and no particular direction.

Nearly a year went by in this fashion before another crisis erupted in Ms. H.'s life. When a friend at work "forgot" a planned luncheon date, Ms. H. experienced a reappearance of the acute anxiety and other symptoms that brought her into treatment originally. Uncharacteristically, she telephoned for an extra appointment, apologizing profusely for this intrusion. When she came in, still tearful and distraught, she seemed quite different. The social worker, for the first time since her original application, experienced her as a "real" client.

After crying several minutes uncontrollably, she stopped herself and said, "I can't do this. This is awful." When the social worker asked why it was awful, she said, "I can't let you see me like this. You must wonder what to do next with me. It must be so draining to listen to people's problems all the time." The social worker pursued this dynamic in subsequent sessions. At another point, Ms. H. said, "I wanted to be your easiest client—someone you'd look forward to. I wanted to give you a chance to sit back and rest—to take a break from all the troubles you have to listen to and carry around." When asked what might happen if she risked burdening the worker with her own feelings, she declared, "You might get overwhelmed and just stop listening!" The social worker wondered, "You mean I might go away? Doesn't this feel familiar?" Ms. H. nodded slowly and cried more profusely than she had done at any other point in their work.

This sequence became a turning point in the treatment. Slowly Ms. H. and the social worker reconstructed that she believed that her parents had been "taken away" because she had been too demanding and needy. She apparently learned early to disguise her neediness from other caregivers and, with praise for her precocity, became a capable caregiver to others as a way of getting her own needs met vicariously. As treatment proceeded, Ms. H. gained access to a broad range of feelings, including fear, loneliness, anger, competitiveness—and a playful sense of humor. Sometimes after reporting a distressing week or an expression of intense affect, she would say, teasingly, "Are you still there?" This capacity to tolerate and try out her "true" self appeared to emerge from the experience of finding out that the social worker could attend to and survive her distress even if she were not his "easiest" client.

Ms. H.'s social worker had been lulled into accepting the respite she wanted to afford him each week. Horner (1979) notes that an overly positive response to the false self may lead the client to assume that the true self would not be welcomed. Supervision is helpful in keeping the treatment effort focused on helping the client be "real."

THE FALSE SELF BUILT ON IDENTIFICATIONS

Further along Winnicott's continuum toward health is the false self built on identifications. Here there is a sense of a distinct, personal self, but it is modeled in an exaggerated way on the behaviors of others rather than being flexibly expressive of the spontaneous true self. This may appear quite normally in adolescence as young people "try on" various identities on the road to consolidation of the true self. But as a persistent life pattern, such identification can stultify psychosocial growth. As Horner (1979) suggests, in this developmental configuration, "there is an established sense of 'I am,' but the elaboration of that self and its characteristics becomes channeled and rigidified along the lines of identifications rather than representing the unfolding patterns more intrinsic to the child himself" (pp. 64–65). Often people who carry this vulnerability into adulthood are able to find relationships in which their essential dependency on others for self-definition is legitimated and supported.

> Mr. O., a 70-year-old man, was referred to a hospital social service department for help in discharge planning for his wife who had suffered a stroke. Mrs. O.'s physician had recommended a period of care in an inpatient rehabilitation facility. As the worker discussed this plan with Mr. O., she became aware of his inability to engage with her in considering options in his community. When asked about his feelings, he began to weep. He told the worker that he could not face the prospect of his wife being away from home for an extended period of time. His daily routine was built around her—getting up to make her coffee, eating meals when she cooked them, consulting with her before he planned an activity for himself. Without her he felt incapable of making any decisions: "When it comes to eating, I can't even shop because I don't know what I feel like eating." As Mr. N. reflected on his life he realized, "I've never had to think for myself. My wife always complained that I didn't start my own business, but the thought of that scared me—all those decisions. And what if I made the wrong ones? Even as a kid, I wasn't expected to think for myself. My mother used to say, 'Just remember, your dad and I have been around a lot longer than you have. We know what's best.' In a way I believed her, but other times I wished she could have had more confidence in some of my ideas. Now it's too late—I don't seem to have any ideas of my own."

Attention to false self elements can be helpful in situations like Mr. N.'s, where a major trauma or loss reveals unevenness in true self development that has been concealed in a relationship where identification with an overfunctioning partner picks up the slack. Differential assessment is crucial in finding out whether a client's indecisiveness is part of a false self or rather results from a temporary failure of normally effective ego functions and defenses.

THE SOCIAL FALSE SELF

Finally, in health the false self finds expression in "the whole organization of the polite and mannered social attitude" (Winnicott 1960b, p. 143). Here we find the appropriate reserve that lends structure and civility to social intercourse. As Grolnick (1990) points out, "without a false self, or in healthy terms, a social self, a true self would never be able to survive in the world" (p. 71). Part of the role of the false self at this adaptive level is legitimate sequestering of the core of true self experience. Ultimately, Winnicott traced with his true and false self concepts a developmental line based on an ongoing dialectic in everyone between the social self and this true, private self—an extension of the developmental dialectic between experiences of connectedness to and separateness from others. Through paying attention to this dialectic, "a therapist can have a good start learning how to offer the patient an ebb and flow of empathy, dissonance, and daring mixed with the ability to hold back and wait" (Grolnick 1990, p. 74).

As Winnicott (1960b) noted, in health a certain degree of false self is present in all relationships, and this naturally includes the clinical relationship. A certain social facade, structured in terms of starting and ending times, a designated place of meeting, fees, and other arrangements of professional exchange, characterizes the clinical interchange. Social worker and client observe the customs and proprieties of social intercourse; sessions may begin with a comment about the weather, for example, or end with client's wish that the worker enjoy a pleasant week. Both worker and client remain aware, however, that at the heart of the clinical relationship lies a space for the expression of the client's true self. Any excessive distraction from this agenda can represent the worker's collusion with the client to avoid exploration of the true self and its associated affects. The social worker can set the stage for clients' comfort in expressing true self elements by taking initiative at the beginning of treatment to state explicitly that they do not have to maintain a false self facade in the clinical relationship. In response to a client's apology for crying or expressing anger, for example, a simple "that's allowed here" can offer permission for the true self to emerge.

It is important to acknowledge, however, that many agencies, especially those where receipt of benefits or services depends on conformity to specific conditions and regulations, reinforce compliance and suppression of the true self in clients. Sometimes there is unspoken awareness on the part of both clients and service professionals that clients are playing along with a service plan, but have no intention of carrying it out as mandated. More insidious are instances where clients learn to feign compliance with authoritarian agencies as a way of obtaining concrete services. Because they do not become engaged in an authentic helping relationship, they unwittingly undermine services that might be of more benefit in preventing further difficulties in their lives. The most carefully developed service plans can be sabotaged when clinicians working in child welfare, the court system, or other agencies where authority and power are at issue fail to attend to this reinforced false self dynamic.

On a broader level, many people have learned to adopt a socially sanctioned false self presentation as a way to survive hostile conditions. Many people of color, women, gays and lesbians, and other oppressed groups have been rewarded for compliance and have had to suppress true self expression in order to deal with the threat of humiliation and harm. Many children of color, for example, learn early to develop a dual identity—one indigenous to their immediate family and ethnic context and another designed to be acceptable to the prevailing white majority. It is crucial to recognize that this false-self behavior is a manifestation of social rather than individual psychopathology, and is often a sign of adaptive skill, strength, and creativity.

An African-American doorman at a large high-income condominium building told his social worker that he was a "totally different person" at work. There he was "George"—polite, attentive, always smiling. At home he was "Mr. Carlton," block captain, highly respected for his leadership skills and his ability to mediate neighborhood disputes. Mr. Carlton attended college in the evenings and he hoped to become a teacher. He sought counseling for a driving phobia after a car accident. He approached a specific social worker who had an office in the building because she had asked his name and always addressed him as "Mr. Carlton." He resented that, while the name on his jacket said "George," he was required to address everyone at work as Mr., Ms., or Doctor. With a resigned shrug he said, "There's no way I can change that in the position I'm in now. I need the money. But when I'm a teacher I'll be respected on the job and everybody will call me Mr. Carlton. For now, at least *I* know who I am."

Only through concentrated policy initiatives toward social justice and civil rights can facilitating environments for true self expression and dignity be realized. Clinical social workers must take these structural issues into account when working with individual clients and view part of their professional role as working politically toward large-scale social change.

PART III

BROADER
IMPLICATIONS

THE GOOD-ENOUGH
SOCIAL WORKER

Attention to contextual aspects of people's lives has always distinguished social work's approach from that of other helping professions. The consistent emphasis on the person-in-environment as the focus of understanding and intervening with individuals, families, groups, and communities has been key to the evolution of a unique social work epistemology. We believe that Winnicott's concept of the potential space between person and environment as the location of cultural experience—and the metaphorical location in which context-responsive intervention takes place—lends new depth and precision to this focus.

Winnicott drew his view of culture from his concept of transitional relatedness, suggesting that cultural life is "the adult equivalent of the transitional phenomena of infancy and early childhood" (1963a, p. 184). Culture can be located, he believed, in the "space" between inner and outer reality, the area originally bridged by the transitional object. Just as the symbolic function of the transitional object both joins and separates infant and caregiver, the potential space of culture both joins people to the larger common pool of humanity and offers a dependable holding environment in which they can realize their potential as individuals.

For Winnicott (1968a), culture was a collective culmination of natural individual growth processes—"a superimposition of a thousand million patterns, the one upon the other" (p. 151). He suggested that people live in three dimensions: the world of the intrapsychic, the world of external reality, and the world of cultural experience in which each person's intrapsychic reality transacts with aspects of external reality. It is in this third dimension that external aspects of culture meet with each person's unique mental representations of culture. And this is the interpersonal space of clinical work—the intermediate area in which social workers can balance an appreciation of individual psychodynamics and perceptions with an appreciation of external aspects of sociocultural diversity. In an increasingly multicultural society, we need to be well acquainted with both.

The potential space metaphor provides a way of naming the dynamic intersystemic arena of social work intervention in which aspects of external reality transact dialectically with each person's subjective construction of that reality. It is this idea that we have attempted to illustrate in the book's varied case examples of agency-based practice.

Each of these examples portrays the kinds of interventions that social workers undertake routinely in their work. We tackle the most challenging problems and, borrowing selectively and prudently from a wide range of social and behavioral theories, marshal our creativity to adapt these theories to the cluttered and unpredictable realities we encounter. As noted earlier, much of what we do is undergirded by the silent, supportive, relationship-based functions that, because they are difficult to name, have tended to be viewed as less refined and rigorous than the interpretive, expressive techniques associated with more traditional psychotherapies. Our difficulty in finding language for this supportive, sustaining activity has played a part in the marginalization of social work among the helping professions—a marginalization that has resulted in lower status and lower pay for our extremely demanding work. We look at the concepts emphasized in this book as additional tools for naming more precisely, and therefore privileging, these crucial but underappreciated activities. We reprise them here to articulate the links between Winnicott's contributions and enduring social work principles, values, and practices. In addition, we consider cultural and other contextual variables that influence assessment and intervention.

THE KEY CONCEPTS REVISITED: CULTURE AND CONTEXT

Central to the full range of social work services is consistent attention to the *holding environment*, from the micro to the macro level. Beyond consideration of a specific client's family, we look at the neighborhood, community, and other larger systems in the client's world in terms of the extent to which they "hold" him or her, or, as is the case with many poorer clients, may have traumatized or "dropped" him or her. Moreover, we evaluate social policies and programs in relation to their holding potential and, where necessary, take steps to change them.

   In applying the holding environment metaphor to the clinical relationship, it is important to distinguish the way caregivers hold infants from the application of supportive interventions. It is not that we infantilize clients by trying to reparent them and make up for earlier caregivers' failures; rather, clinical "holding" means that we afford clients the same level of respectful, individualized attention that good-enough caregivers afford their infants. Failure to make this distinction can be deleterious. Fantasies that we should or can rescue or repair clients may unwittingly lead us to absolve them from responsibility for changing themselves and their situations, thus subtly disempowering them. Holding is a useful metaphor for intervention, but applied literally it does not do justice to the nuanced complexities of effective supportive work.

Clearly, the immediate holding environment of earliest infancy is the family, but as clinician-scholars like Carter and McGoldrick (1989) suggest, the formation and composition of the family varies widely across and within cultures. They point out that for many first-generation Italians, for example, the tripartite nuclear family may not exist. Instead, family consists of a complex and extensive network of aunts, uncles, cousins, and grandparents who often live, if not in the same dwelling, in close proximity. Many African-American families go beyond blood relatives to include a range of friends and church affiliates in their definition of family (Stack 1975). In many Mexican-American and Puerto Rican families, an elaborate godparent system assures the availability of several parent substitutes to the developing child (Martinez 1988, Ramos-McKay et al. 1988). In these and other diverse family configurations encountered by social workers, the holding environment concept expands to include culture.

Winnicott's concept of *ego relatedness* adds new language to social work's discourse on the value of the helping relationship. This concept reminds us that "there is no such thing as a client"—rather it is the collaborative, facilitating partnership between worker and client that acts as the catalyst for change. The idea of ego relatedness does not negate the importance to human functioning of instinctual drives, conflicts, defenses, and other aspects of intrapsychic life. But, it focuses our attention on the strivings for relatedness and connectedness that, as recent research on infants confirms, are operational and motivational from birth. The emphasis here is on the "self-in-relation" and on the importance of being able to have a sense of psychological well-being in the intimate presence of others as well as in solitude.

The nature of ego relatedness will, of course, be influenced by the variations in family composition described above. In family and kinship systems where multiple caregivers are available, the extended group of alternative "objects" can serve as a "secondary protective barrier" from external impingements (Panel 1968, p. 658). Muensterberger (Panel 1968) suggests that the availability and interchangeability of several caregivers leads to the development of mental representations of caregiving functions that are more diffuse than those of infants cared for primarily by one or two people.

Ego relatedness is also shaped by specific child-rearing practices and their associated values. Because human infants experience a lengthy period of physical dependence, cultural provisions for their protection appear universally. There is wide variation, however, in the manner in which families orchestrate this protection. This variation arises from diverse beliefs and practices related to childbirth as well as from culturally determined views about the nature and purpose of development. Western conceptions of development, for example, tend to view infants as undifferentiated, highly dependent beings who must be drawn from symbiosis toward independence from others. People in many Eastern cultures, in contrast, see infants as separate and differentiated from birth and in need of being drawn increasingly into interdependence with others (Caudill and Weinstein 1969). As noted earlier, recent studies of infants suggest that their internal experiences oscillate dialectically between feelings of oneness with and separateness from others (Kaplan 1987). The side of the dialectic that receives emphasis in the understanding of development, however, varies culturally. Because they influence the manner in which individuals nurture and interact with their infants, resulting cultural practices ultimately shape childrens' object relations. They remap intrapsychic and interpersonal potential space.

In attending to the *transitional process*, social workers acknowledge and support the ways in which clients form and use attachments to both human and non-human "objects" as they find creative avenues to self-soothing in stressful contexts. The transitional object concept offers a way to conceptualize the importance of people's attachments to agencies, institutions, programs, and ideologies. With this concept, we have a way to think about the importance of religion and spirituality to clients and to incorporate this understanding in plans for assisting them. This idea also offers a way to think about sociocultural diversity as an aspect of transitional "space" between worker and client that can be bridged through sensitive inquiry.

Varying conceptions of family, development, and associated child-rearing practices inevitably influence expressions of transitional relatedness. The popularity of Winnicott's (1953) transitional object concept has led to its becoming a routine focus of inquiry in developmental history-taking and other aspects of assessment. In general, a child's attachment to transitional objects and phenomena is viewed as an indicator of psychological health, whereas an absence or atypical use of them is associated with psychopathology. But the database for this perspective emerges primarily from observational research on small samples of white, middle-class children in nursery schools operated by child study centers or university departments and from case-study reports of remembered attachments as reported by children and adults in psychoanalytic psychotherapy. The danger of generalizing from this narrowly defined cohort lies in the potential attribution of pathology to behavior that may be normal when placed in context.

Applegate's (1989) review of cross-cultural research on transitional objects and phenomena reveals that the presence or absence of specific transitional objects will vary with family sleeping arrangements, the degree and importance ascribed to holding, rocking, and similar direct physical contact, and the availability and extent of caregiving by extended or surrogate family members. Findings suggest that strong attachments to these objects are more likely to be formed by children growing up in families where they are expected to wean early, sleep alone, and in other ways move toward self-sufficiency at an early age. Transitional object attachments are much less frequent in contexts where children sleep with their parents or siblings, are carried on the mother's back, or in other ways experience extended physical contact and have access to multiple caregivers. Knowledge of such variation helps guide differential assessment and context-responsive intervention.

Winnicott's concept of *object relating and object use* helps us reframe resistance, poor motivation, or a hostile, confrontational posture as an adaptive effort to test the limits and durability of a new, probably anxiety-provoking relationship. Awareness of this concept promotes starting where the client is and enables us to be accepting and nonjudgmental of provocative behavior. Winnicott saw such behavior as a sign that clients have not given up hope that the environment will survive their challenges and respond to them with understanding and support. Depathologizing aggression helps workers to maintain empathy for clients whose defensive agenda may be to keep them at a distance. Both the creativity implied in the concept of the transitional process and the capacity for hope implied in the shift from object relating to object use resonate with social work's respect for clients' strengths and competencies.

It is in the process of moving from object relating to object usage that skin color and other observable manifestations of race and ethnicity appear to play a particularly salient role. Bowles (1988), for example, suggests that attitudes toward racial and ethnic characteristics, like others, are internalized through mirroring interactions and become "ethnic self-representation units" that are encoded and transmitted from generation to generation as enduring mental structures. To the concluding phase of the separation-individuation process described by Mahler, Pine, and Bergman (1975) Bowles adds the attainment of "ethnic object constancy." For African-Americans and other people of color exposed to institutional racism, the provision of interpersonal conditions facilitative of positive ethnic and racial object constancy can be very difficult. When the majority culture views skin color negatively, the developing child may take in negative self and object representations carried by caregivers and communicated in their mirroring behaviors. Evolving from the ambivalence caregivers have internalized toward their own racial characteristics, resulting ego structures may become expressed in a "defensive, affect-laden, questioning attitude about living in the world" (Bowles 1988, p. 110).

Especially in conditions of poverty, where surrounding systems fail to support these families, this attitude may impede object usage. Pinderhughes and her associates (1979) identify several maternal behaviors that, although intended to prepare children of color to live safely in a racist society, have the unintended effect of compromising their capacity to employ healthy aggression in the service of self–object differentiation. The racially oppressed caregiver may try to "toughen up" her child for life in harsh conditions by abrupt handling and an early push toward independence. Resulting feelings of being abandoned or "dropped" may predispose her child to feelings of helplessness and rage that an immature ego is ill equipped to integrate. Or, motivated by the same concern about hostile conditions, the caregiver may cling to the child and become hypervigilant in ways that impede development.

Related to this overprotection is a tendency neither to allow children to take initiative in relationships nor to foster their exploration and manipulation of the environment in the service of discovery and mastery. This curtailment of curiosity and self-assertion evolves from a conviction that "to tolerate the child's emerging aggression is dangerously maladaptive" (Pinderhughes et al. 1979, p. 20). As a result, the appearance of the child's normal aggression may be met with retaliation rather than tolerance. Rather than a galvanizing affect that can be integrated into a positive self-concept and employed in the service of object usage, aggression may be turned either toward the self in the form of resignation and depression or outward toward society in the form of antisocial behavior. Ultimately, such outcomes compromise the development of agency and mastery that are aspects of the true self.

For social workers, the *true and false self* concept speaks to the value of self-determination in its most fundamental sense by fostering interventions that individualize each client and his or her situation toward facilitating the potential, not just for surviving, but for feeling grounded and thoroughly alive. It helps us remember that, regardless of the presenting problem and its seeming urgency, we want to offer in our interventions the opportunity for clients to find and develop their own voices toward personal growth and self-acceptance. The goal is full collaboration in the helping effort, a goal that is often difficult to operationalize with clients like those described above whose racial and/or economic oppression has rendered them understandably suspicious of helping efforts. Such clients may present an overly compliant false-self posture that makes engagement with the true self very difficult.

In addition, some of the policies and procedures in agencies require compliance rather than encourage assertion in clients. Entangled in complicated and restrictive bureaucracies, social workers in such settings can emerge as authoritarian in their approach. Clients, in turn, learn to protect rather than reveal their true selves through apparent obedience, or they may find that the only avenue available for keeping allegiance to their true selves is through dropping out of treatment. Part of the social worker's role in agencies, therefore, is to monitor policies and procedures in terms of their demands for compliance by clients in services that suppress rather than support their right to personal authenticity.

KEEPING THE INDIVIDUAL CLIENT IN MIND

Winnicott's "potential space" metaphor reminds us that, although sociocultural groups and subgroups may hold in common certain generalized representations of self and other, each person's unique early experiences and relationships will lead him or her to ascribe different meanings to cultural and other external factors. As Winnicott (1966) put it, "For the five children in a family there are five families" (p. 132). He might have said the same for culture, race and ethnicity, and social class. The clinical challenge is to find a way to consider simultaneously the sociocultural factors in people's lives while addressing their idiosyncratic interpretations of these factors. Saari (1994) suggests that the capacity for empathy that makes true individualization possible depends on the social worker's ability to move back and forth cognitively between his or her own sociocultural context and that of the client. Extending Winnicott's ideas about culture and the transitional process, Saari coins the phrase "playing in transcontextual space" to describe the process of developing and sustaining clinical empathy for clients whose heritage differs from that of the worker.

Recognizing that each individual "creates" his or her own experience of culture on the basis of idiosyncratic self and object representations, clinicians can set up therapeutic conditions where yet another culture can develop—the new culture formed in the shared reality of the therapeutic relationship (Saari 1986). This culture will generate its own customs, rituals, language, and organizing metaphors. In the quietly alive potential or "transcontextual" space between clinician and client, we can listen for the impact of diversity while avoiding stereotypic assumptions that may or may not apply to specific clients. Beyond this private sphere of influence, social workers have a responsibility to intervene toward social change. Broader expressions of a capacity for concern include advocacy, political organizing, opposition to institutionalized racism, sexism, and homophobia, as well as other efforts to alter oppressive social conditions.

BEYOND DIRECT PRACTICE

A quarter century ago Winnicott (1969) advised:

> Social workers need just now to look at the philosophy of their work all the time; they need to know when they must fight to be allowed (and paid) to do the difficult and not the easy thing; they must find support where it can be found and not expect support from administration. In fact . . . social workers need to be themselves the parent figures, sure of their own attitude even when unsupported and often in the curious position of claiming the right to be worn out in the exercise of their duties, rather than to be seduced into the easy way of inducing conformity. [p. 559]

How can the profession prepare social workers to heed Winnicott's impassioned call for self-definition, self-advocacy, and pride in their work?

EDUCATION AND TRAINING

Since its inception, the social work profession has viewed the helping relationship as the bedrock of practice. Through decades of experience with clients and social systems presenting the most challenging of human difficulties, social workers have learned to take the centrality of the relationship for granted. Recently, however, there has been a trend in social work education away from a focus on the relationship and toward training for specific techniques. Frequently derived from behavioral and cognitive approaches, these interventions are easier to quantify and, therefore, appear to be better suited to research methods designed to measure treatment outcome (Hanna 1993).

There is little question that social workers must continue to develop methods that help them document the effectiveness of their work. The current fiscal climate of diminished funding and escalating insurance and other health care costs makes such documentation a necessity. But approaches to inquiry and education that de-emphasize the role of the relationship in clinical work leave students ill-equipped for the real world of practice. Some students are placed in field agencies that urge them to make assessments and treatment plans quickly, often after one session. These students learn how to gather histories and other psychosocial data with facility. And, drawing on a growing store of empirically based intervention techniques, they quickly learn to design and measure task-focused treatment strategies. But closer examination of their work reveals that they have little sense of how to build a relationship—or even how to comfortably "be" with their clients. They are puzzled when their treatment plans fail, clients drop out prematurely, or, after a sense that the tasks were completed and the problem solved, clients reappear in the throes of a new crisis. Scrutiny of the case often reveals that key relationship dynamics have been overlooked and that the treatment has floundered due to a failure to attend to them.

Winnicott's concepts offer students a frame of reference and an accessible language for keeping the helping relationship in the spotlight, regardless of the nature of the intervention. Beginners develop a sense of what a therapeutic holding environment is and how to make clients feel safe and comfortable. They incorporate the concepts of ego and transitional relatedness, and grasp their possible role as a transitional object for a troubled family. They can learn to become attuned to clients' spontaneous gestures and can understand that an angry outburst has meaning beyond its literal expression, thus finding theoretical support for the therapeutic value of "surviving" such an outburst.

The basis for such understanding of client behavior and relationship building derives from developmental theory that can be incorporated into foundation courses in Human Behavior and the Social Environment. In such a course, taught by one of the authors for several years, students have found Winnicott's concepts to be both theoretically illuminating and useful in practice. As noted earlier in the book, Winnicott's concepts are epistemologically congruent with systems or ecological theory, increasingly the basis for many texts used in human behavior courses. While an appreciation of the multiple external systems within which clients transact their lives is crucial, a knowledge of the intra- and interpsychic systems within which they develop is also essential. Such knowledge helps students to appreciate the complexity of human development and behavior and to individualize clients by appreciating how each person will bring his or her own unique perceptions to troubling life events and circumstances.

Winnicott's ideas can also be incorporated into beginning and advanced practice courses in schools of social work. They help students to grasp the importance of establishing a therapeutic holding environment for clients as part of initial engagement and to appreciate the importance of preserving this safe interpersonal haven through the subsequent phases of assessment, intervention, and termination. Details of relationship building are amplified through attention to the concept of ego relatedness, and students can recognize points in the intervention when clients are developing a capacity to make use of them and of the agency as transitional objects. The dynamics of transference, counter-transference, and resistance can be examined in terms of the developmental move from object relating to object use. When students begin to grasp that, despite their most caring efforts, clients may subjectively conceive of them as depriving, demanding, or abandoning, this frame of reference helps them to remain empathic and endure the testing that may usher in clients' capacity to view them more objectively as resources for growth. Finally, the recognition of the client's right to true self determination will enable beginning clinicians to celebrate rather than retaliate against clients' assertive efforts to claim themselves.

Some educators believe that psychodynamic concepts and practice approaches are lost on clients whose social circumstances are so depriving or oppressive as to keep them in a perpetual state of acute need or crisis. Certainly environmental modification, advocacy, and the provision of concrete services are essential in many such situations. But humane service delivery demands that attention be paid to the *meaning* clients ascribe to their trying situations and to services provided to assist them.

Examination of meaning requires attention to the dynamics of the helping relationship. Sometimes an assumption is made that, due to a lack of education, an absence of psychological-mindedness, or underdeveloped verbal skills, many social work clients cannot benefit from psychodynamic approaches. We contend that this assumption constitutes a subtle but pernicious form of discrimination and oppression. In fact, often it is those who have been most deprived, abused, or neglected who most benefit from an approach that includes a dynamic understanding of their dilemmas. Such clients often respond positively and deeply to someone who is willing to sit quietly with them, to listen to their own version of their story, to attempt to help them find meaning in the predicaments in their lives. This approach is the essence of a *facilitating* partnership—one designed to set into motion the reparative tendency that social workers have long recognized to be extant in every human being. When clients can begin to understand that their crises have antecedents in their past situations and relationships, they are empowered to begin to make changes in previously maladaptive patterns. And when they begin to understand that the clinician will not respond to them or their situations as others from their past may have, they can make use of the new relationship to chart a new course.

SUPERVISION

For both students and more seasoned social workers, this approach can be nurtured through clinical supervision. As noted, many clients seen by social workers cannot easily formulate or verbalize their feelings. Clinicians have to develop empathic understanding primarily through the medium of their countertransference reactions. Making use of one's own subjective responses in this way implies having access to a professionally useable inner life (Saari 1990). Access to this inner life is facilitated by "the maintenance of a receptive space for the arrival of news from within the self" (Bollas 1987, p. 239). This news from within most frequently emerges as a feeling state of "not-knowing-yet-experiencing" (p. 203). Bollas asserts further that "The capacity to bear and value this necessary uncertainty defines one of our most important clinical responsibilities" (p. 203). Through not knowing, the worker keeps the potential space of clinical work open so as to learn how the client may be "using" him or her. Feelings of depletion, depression, sexual arousal, rage, detachment—all these may be clues to what the client is asking the clinician to contain and, thus, know indirectly.

To hear and make therapeutic use of countertransference news from within, the clinician must be able to differentiate between those feelings arising from his or her own unique relational history or current stresses and those being generated primarily by the client's projections and projective identifications. Supervision that includes a focus on the worker's countertransference reactions can help the worker disentangle his or her own issues from those of the clients. Often, a social worker under pressure by a client to "do something" will turn to supervision for advice or guidance—a call for the supervisor to tell him or her what to do, thus replicating the unconscious elements of the client–worker interaction. Responding to these injunctions to action, the "good-enough supervisor" works to preserve the potential space for reflective consideration of the client's issues and corresponding countertransference reactions in the worker. The supervisor's role in these instances is neither to make suggestions nor offer reassurance, but rather "to allow the emotional disturbance to be felt within the safer setting of the supervisory relationship, where it can be survived, reflected upon and learnt from" (Hawkins and Shohet 1989, p. 3). Such abstinence requires the supervisor to be able to bear the anxiety and depression aroused by the supervisee's most difficult cases. As part of this process, the supervisor may model reflective practice by refraining from talking too much or in other ways violating the potential space of supervision. By providing periods in supervision where the supervisee is left "alone" in this way, the supervisor helps him or her develop the capacity to be alone in the presence of the client (Yerushalmi 1992). This capacity helps create the potential space for the eventual presence of what Casement (1991) calls the "internal supervisor"—the internalized aspects of supervision that become part of the supervisee's object world and act as an ongoing holding environment. Winnicottian supervision is likely to be enhanced by the social worker's own therapy, a valuable, indeed essential, adjunct to training for this type of work.

REFLECTIVE INQUIRY AND
KNOWLEDGE BUILDING

Social work practice guided by a Winnicottian framework is congruent with the current thrust in the profession toward narrative and other constructivist approaches to research and theory development (see Dean 1989, 1993, Gorman 1993). As noted earlier, Winnicott's own way of developing ideas about theory and practice presaged this recent hermeneutic turn. Rather than make efforts to interpret or explain away uncertainty, he embraced it as an opportunity to explore the "unthought known" (Bollas 1987) of clients' inner worlds. He focused in his practice on setting up conditions in which clients could reveal their true selves through direct experience in the clinical relationship. He was interested in the client's story as co-constructed in the matrix of this relationship—whether that story was told in the form of a mutually executed squiggle drawing, a dream, transference and countertransference reactions, or in verbal discourse. Instead of an expert ready to translate what the client presented into an interpretation, Winnicott positioned himself as a curious listener trying to understand another's story in order to more sensitively co-author a new story more facilitative of the client's potential. Building on his example, we can become curious students open to learning from the client about the unique personal, social, and cultural determinants of his or her situation. Through the medium of the combined ingredients of the client's story and the worker's efforts to make meaning of it (the worker's theories), new meaning systems are created. Saleebey (1994) captures this approach succinctly: "So with clients, we act as collaborators, cofacilitators, and codirectors as we work to resurrect, confirm, or disconfirm old meanings; establish 'better texts'; and, most importantly, discover how different meanings differently influence people's lives" (p. 357).

This approach requires a broadening of the scope and methods of social work's research agenda to include a place for what Winnicott (1965b) referred to as the search for "poetic truth"—the truth that "is a matter of feeling [about which] we may not all feel the same" (p. 172). Winnicott had great respect for the modernist scientific tradition of technical rationality in which he was schooled, with its focus on objectivity, quantification, and prediction. But his belief that "science boggles at the problem of human nature, and tends to lose sight of the whole human being" (1965, p. 173) reveals his essential postmodern leanings. Capturing the experience of the whole human being calls for research derived from a variety of ways of knowing, both nomothetic and idiographic, quantitative and qualitative. It makes a place for studies that explore mimetic knowledge—knowledge grounded in and derived from bodily awareness (Saleebey 1989)—as well as intellectually derived knowledge. A broadened definition of research makes a place for inquiry that includes studies of narrative texts of interventions and looks at case studies as stories whose authenticity or truth speaks for itself and needn't be generalized to other clinical experiences.

Through these and other qualitative methods of telling social work's stories, we open doors for new research possibilities. Among the most promising of these possibilities is the practice of writing as a form of inquiry. Reading Winnicott conveys the sense that he used writing as a research tool, constantly exploring and re-exploring clinical and theoretical concepts through the medium of his considerable written oeuvre. His writing is ellipitcal and opaque, yet intuitively engaging and accessible. The reader has the experience of "knowing" what he means but not quite grasping the meaning conceptually. Winnicott played with the words of others to explore what they meant to him; thus, for example, he transforms Klein's concept of the depressive position to the more experience-near, less pathologizing, "capacity for concern."

Such experiences of discovery and reinvention are captured in Richardson's (1994) description of the way she employs writing as a way of knowing, a method of discovery and analysis: "I write because I want to find something out. I write in order to learn something that I didn't know before I wrote it" (p. 517). As Richardson sees it, writing-as-inquiry need not be limited to the conventions of the traditional research report but can take more experimental forms, including drama, poetry, and short stories. Winnicott's own written record is punctuated by snippets of poetry, imaginative essays, and letters that express his developing ideas in different forms. With increasing support in the profession for postmodern approaches to inquiry, social workers can be encouraged to write about their day-to-day work in innovative ways that generate practice knowledge for themselves as well as their readers.

SOCIAL POLICIES AND PROGRAMS

As is true for all social workers, the professional responsibilities of the Winnicottian social worker extend beyond the office and the agency. Securing facilitating environments for people requires sustained social action and other forms of influence at the levels of policy and program development, implementation, and support. Winnicott offers us a model for such an extension of his theories to the public arena; along with his wife Clare, he was a tireless social advocate. His activities included vigorous letter writing campaigns to public officials about inequities in child and family mental health policy, letters to newspaper editors taking stands against what he viewed as inhumane treatment of people with major mental illness, and spirited talks to child care workers, teachers, corrections officers, and others responsible for the well-being of children and families (see Rodman 1987, Winnicott 1984, C. Winnicott et al. 1989).

The implications of Winnicott's ideas for prevention and policy are obvious. His theories support what social workers have known since the inception of the profession. Social policies and programs that provide the basics of food, clothing, shelter, and adequate medical care for every individual are imperative. These are the linchpins for an adequate social holding environment, the fundamental prerequisites for an individual and community sense of going-on-being. Comprehensive prenatal care is also crucial, not only in monitoring the expectant mother's health but in helping her attend to and become emotionally preoccupied with her unborn child. Prepared childbirth is another avenue for fostering relatedness to the expected baby and, whenever possible, should include the father. When fathers can be engaged at this early stage in the birth process there is a greater likelihood that they will want to take their place in the new baby's holding environment and be available as another object for ego relatedness (Applegate 1987).

Early postnatal care should also be a basic provision, both to monitor the health of the nursing couple and to begin to address any relational misattunements resulting from differences in temperament between mother and infant. Very early intervention can assist caregivers in tuning-in to the unique personal styles of their infants and in altering their holding, handling, and object presenting accordingly. Programs that attend to these emotional issues are as important as those that attend to the infant's physical health. Only equal attention to both aspects of development assures the integration of psyche and soma that fosters a feeling of aliveness in babies and promotes the evolution of the true self.

Winnicott's theory points to the preventive efficacy of parenting programs that can inform and support parents at all stages of their children's development. Such programs may include but must go beyond parent education. If carefully designed on the basis of a developmental perspective, these programs provide a safe interpersonal space wherein parents can discuss the range of affective responses their babies evoke in them. Assisted in verbalizing the range of their feelings, parents can consider them reflectively in a way that may prevent acting them out. As they learn that it is normal periodically to be irked by—even periodically to hate—their children (see Winnicott 1993), they gain greater tolerance for their children's periodic need to "destroy" them in the service of individuation.

As both parents in increasing numbers of families enter the full-time work force, affordable, high-quality day care becomes essential. As noted earlier, the exclusive mother–infant bond is no longer the norm in our society; it is clear from infant research and from cross-cultural studies that babies can become productively attached to a variety of caregivers. It is not so much the person of the mother but the *maternal provision* that emerges as crucial.

Fundamental to this provision are consistency and reliability—qualities that are sorely missing from many day-care programs. The extent to which we as a society undervalue the need for day care is reflected in the low payscales of child care workers. Also, administrators may ask personnel to look after too many children, thus depriving all of them of individual attention. Underpaid and overworked, many child care workers stay at their jobs only briefly. Children in these circumstances are asked to deal with repeated cycles of brief attachment and loss—loss which, depending on their age, may be experienced as abandonment. Because their reactions to these losses often go unrecognized, they may act out their feelings in disruptive ways, thus further distancing and frustrating the staff. A commitment to social justice and the support of families—especially families of poverty—requires making funding for day care a national policy priority.

In situations where conditions require placing children in ongoing care outside their families of origin, reliability and consistency again are the mainstays of successful placement. In too many child welfare programs, services are fragmented among various personnel. How are children and families to achieve psychosocial integration when services designed for them are disintegrated? In some cases, foster care services, mental health services, financial support services, and others are each represented by different personnel. Children and families in these situations have little opportunity to form a relationship with one consistent person or team to assure a sense of going-on-being in an otherwise chaotic world. It is the growing recognition of this need for consistency and continuity that has given rise to programs that make comprehensive care the responsibility of one individual or small team. In this approach, social workers are assigned a manageably small number of families and are responsible for coordinating the full range of services that a given family may require. By fostering ego relatedness to one or two people, this approach reduces clients' sense of fragmentation, minimizes delays, duplication of services, and bureaucratic mix-ups, and in other ways promotes a sense of cohesion and organization in the service of the holding environment.

In regard to early education, Winnicott (1965b) asserted that "Teachers need to be introduced to the dynamics of infant and child care as much as they need to be taught what to teach" (p. 179). He believed that teachers equipped with a knowledge of these dynamics can set up facilitating environments for creative learning rather than authoritarian environments in which the focus is on depositing static facts into children's minds. Teachers, like parents, need classroom environments that can become "potential spaces" wherein children's spontaneous gestures can be perceived and welcomed and in which ideas can be played with. And in education, as in parenting, holding is composed of a balance between nurturant support and firm limit setting. This approach calls for sensitivity to individual children's needs and requires, therefore, small classrooms, adequate educational supplies, and administrative support. Head Start programs have successfully incorporated these prerequisites and should be a funding priority.

It is important to note that cycles of developmental vulnerability can also occur as the result of trauma in families otherwise "held" securely by society's larger systems. Winnicott believed that all human beings who are subject to major disruptions in the sense of going-on-being at any point can experience unbearable agonies. In a wide variety of settings, social workers encounter people in crisis whose ego functions and defenses have been assaulted, who feel dropped into unfamiliar and frightening circumstances.

Children facing surgery, for example, can better tolerate the trauma if as much of their familiar holding environment as possible can be kept intact. The increasingly popular practice of making arrangements for parents to "room-in" with their children speaks to this need. Children also profit from opportunities to play out, talk about, or otherwise process the meaning of what's happening to them. Such interventions not only help minimize the child's anxiety at the time but also serve a preventive purpose. If unprocessed, the fears and anxieties attendant to violation of the child's body integrity can be split-off and "stored" in the psyche, leading to later nightmares, separation panic, acting out, and other symptoms of unresolved distress.

Surprisingly few settings provide in-depth psychological help to children in medical settings. Moreover, the reactions of their parents and other caregivers are frequently overlooked or misunderstood. Sometimes little more is required than a social worker's asking the parents, "How are *you* doing?" or "What is this like for you?" Yet in many instances known to both authors, families are contacted by social service personnel only in relation to insurance arrangements, discharge planning, or as the result of their specific requests. Families in shock over the illness or accident of a loved one are often too overwhelmed to process information being communicated by medical personnel. The presence of someone to listen with them and to review the information and its meaning to them can have a positive impact on the entire treatment process. In this and other stressful situations where families must navigate unfamiliar, technically complex settings, social workers can become transitional objects who provide a sense of continuity and stability. With such assistance, families are helped to sustain a "primary preoccupation" with the emotional and relational needs of the ill relative.

Social workers know the value of such activities, but the fiscal priorities of today's medical care become impediments to carrying them out. With Diagnosis Related Groupings (DRGs) and other aspects of managed health care, the focus can shift easily from the therapeutic relationship to the mechanics of concrete planning for discharge that distances workers from the family's current needs. This altered focus separates rather than joins helpers and those who need their help. The resulting estrangement is detrimental to families and contributes to burnout in social workers, who begin to see themselves as detached technicians rather than engaged clinicians.

None of the foregoing is new—we know what children and families need and continue to struggle at the micro and the macro levels of intervention for social conditions that promote equity, justice, and psychological well-being. We believe, however, that Winnicott's theories offer especially potent and convincing concepts with which social workers can build and support their arguments. These concepts are both theoretically well-grounded and have broad intuitive appeal.

MANAGED CARE

Current efforts to rescue and transform America's ailing health care system present new challenges and threats to good social work practice. Nowhere are these challenges more apparent than in the current trend toward managed care in the delivery of mental health services. In efforts to curtail the costs of psychotherapy and other mental health services, insurance companies and health plans are stepping over the boundaries of the helping relationship to regulate its parameters and duration. The thrust of managed mental health care is toward rapid assessment and brief intervention, overseen by a representative of the external funding source who must approve the intervention plan and any extensions of service beyond the minimum number of sessions required for basic symptom relief. From behind the scenes, these reviewers not only determine the extent of clients' benefits and the clinician's level of compensation; they evaluate the clinician's performance as well, threatening to deny future referrals if treatment is prolonged (Alperin 1994). Such an arrangement constitutes an impingement on the holding environment of the therapeutic relationship and, therefore, is antithetical to many types of intensive intervention—especially those based on psychodynamic principles. As noted earlier, effective supervision eventuates in the supervisee's introjection of a supportive, nonintrusive, "internal supervisor" (Casement 1991) whose capacity to bear uncertainty and reflect on the vicissitudes of countertransference prepares the clinician for empathic practice with challenging clients. Managed care, in contrast, imposes foreign "external supervisors" whose lack of knowledge about and affective distance from the intra- and interpsychic complexity of the case renders them impervious to the impact of their management strategies on the clinician and on the therapeutic relationship (Alperin 1994). The social worker's primary preoccupation shifts from establishing ego relatedness to concern about documenting the necessity for and validity of his or her work. There is pressure for the worker to comply with the reviewer's agenda, thus setting up conditions in which the worker presents a false-self posture to the funding company while attempting to preserve authenticity within the clinical relationship. Clients sense such disjunctures in ways that restrict their full participation in the helping effort.

Managed care's requirement of frequent documentation of the need for ongoing treatment imposes a particularly troublesome impediment to all in-depth clinical work. Organizations that require notes of each session violate confidentiality. Subjecting the most intimate details of the client's inner life to outside scrutiny destroys trust and inhibits clients from sharing with their social workers the very thoughts, feelings, and fantasies that trouble them most. Certainly, not all such work need be long-term: many of the case examples in this book describe interventions that succeeded in one or a few sessions. And some of Winnicott's most compelling case reports depict transformative clinical experiences that occurred in consultations (see, for example, Winnicott 1971f). But there are many instances when longer-term work is essential, especially for the developmentally and materially deprived clients seen in social work settings. What emerges as important is the therapeutic space within which to individualize the length of service according to the client's presenting problems, the extent of the client's developmental or psychological vulnerability, and the way in which he or she makes use of the helping relationship. As Meyer (1993) has argued so convincingly, the "vanishing holding environment" of long-term treatment is a worrisome trend for those who work with clients whose issues demand and deserve extended service.

If viewed through a Winnicottian lens, managed care would take on a more hopeful, less manipulative cast. Describing Winnicott's approach, Khan (1975) notes that "management, in fact, is the provision of that environmental adaptation, in the clinical situation and outside it, which the patient had lacked in his developmental process, and without which all he can do is exist through reactive exploitation of defence mechanisms" (p. xxvii). This approach, while it can inform brief crisis intervention, may require extended periods of time that can allow for the inevitable cycles of regression and progression that accompany effective psychodynamic intervention.

Winnicott also used the metaphor of good-enough caregiving to capture his concept of care. As previously noted, he asserted that "cure at its root means care" (Winnicott 1970a). While we avoid infantalizing clients and cannot care for them literally, we need the therapeutic time and space to become preoccupied with them in a way similar to that which caregivers afford their infants—to listen, hear the client's version fully, and be open to the internal responses the client may evoke in us. This therapeutic accessibility requires flexibility from funding sources and a reevaluation of their bias that briefer is better.

Winnicott's ideas about how people grow and change help us predict what can happen to clients whose treatment does not provide the time and flexibility to attend adequately and sensitively to their own dynamics and to the dynamics of the therapeutic relationship. The amount of money initially saved by managed care restrictions on the length of service is likely to be spent—and often exceeded—later. Inadequate care at the agency level is likely to shift the need for continuing and more expensive care to other institutions: to inpatient units for clients whose under-treated chronic conditions become florid and dangerous; to doctors' offices for stress-induced somatic conditions; to the workplace, where unresolved mental health problems result in increased absenteeism; and to the public sector, which must contend with the financial as well as social costs associated with abuse, neglect, addiction, homelessness, delinquency, and other sequelae of family and societal breakdown. Social workers must take leadership to assure that future health and mental health policy provides for managed care in the truest, Winnicottian sense.

CONCLUSION

Toward the end of his life, Winnicott (1968b) noted that, in his estimation, "the ultimate compliment is to be found and used" (p. 103). It has been our intention to help readers of this book find Winnicott by reviewing his key contributions to psychodynamic theory and by demonstrating how we've applied them in agency-based social work practice. Now it falls to readers to use Winnicott in their own ways, translating his ideas into practice with their own clients in their own work settings. This process of discovery and reinvention constitutes the essence of Winnicott's conception of creativity—a legacy of inspiration and optimism for change that can help sustain our commitment to humane social services into the twenty-first century.

REFERENCES

Abel, T. M., Métraux, R., and Roll, S. (1987). *Psychotherapy and Culture*. Albuquerque, NM: University of New Mexico.

Adler, G. (1977). Hospital management of borderline patients and its relation to psychotherapy. In *Borderline Personality Disorders: The Concept, the Syndrome, the Patient*, ed. P. Hartocollis, pp. 307–323. New York: International Universities Press.

Alperin, R. (1994). Managed care versus psychoanalytic psychotherapy: conflicting ideologies. *Clinical Social Work Journal* 22:137–147.

Anderson, R. (1978). Thoughts on fathering: its relationship to the borderline condition in adolescence and to transitional phenomena. *Adolescent Psychiatry* 6:377–395.

Anzieu, D. (1989). *The Skin Ego: A Psychoanalytic Approach to the Self*. Trans. C. Turner. New Haven, CT: Yale University Press.

Applegate, J. S. (1984). Transitional phenomena in adolescence: tools for negotiating the second individuation. *Clinical Social Work Journal* 12: 233–243.

———— (1987). Beyond the dyad: including the father in separation-individuation. *Child and Adolescent Social Work Journal* 4:92–105.

———— (1989). The transitional object reconsidered: some sociocultural variations and their implications. *Child and Adolescent Social Work Journal* 6:38–51.

———— (1990). Theory, culture, and behavior: object relations in context. *Child and Adolescent Social Work Journal* 7:85–100.

———— (1993). Winnicott and clinical social work: a facilitating partnership. *Child and Adolescent Social Work Journal* 10:3–19.

Applegate, J. S., and Barol, B. I. (1989). Repairing the nest: a psychodynamic developmental approach to clients with severe behavior disorders. *Clinical Social Work Journal* 17:197–207.

Argyris, C. (1980). *The Inner Contradictions of Rigorous Research.* New York: Academic.

Argyris, C., and Schön, D. A. (1974). *Theory in Practice: Increasing Professional Effectiveness.* San Francisco: Jossey-Bass.

Arkema, P. (1981). The borderline personality and transitional relatedness. *American Journal of Psychiatry* 138:172–177.

Barkin, L. (1978). The concept of the transitional object. In *Between Reality and Fantasy: Transitional Objects and Phenomena*, ed. S. A. Grolnick and L. Barkin, pp. 513–536. Northvale, NJ: Jason Aronson.

Benson, R. M. (1980). Narcissistic guardians: developmental aspects of transitional objects, imaginary companions, and career fantasies. In *Adolescent Psychiatry: vol. 3. Developmental and Clinical Studies*, eds. S. L. Feinstein, P. L. Giovacchini, J. C. Looney et al. Chicago: University of Chicago Press.

Berman, L. E. A. (1972). The role of amphetamine in a case of hysteria. *Journal of the American Psychoanalytic Association* 20:325–340.

Bion, W. R. (1962). *Learning from Experience.* New York: Basic Books.

Blanck, G., and Blanck, R. (1979). *Ego Psychology II: Psychoanalytic Developmental Psychology.* New York: Columbia University Press.

Blos, P. (1967). The second individuation process of adolescence.

Psychoanalytic Study of the Child 22:162–186. New York: International Universities Press.

Bollas, C. (1987). *The Shadow of the Object: Psychoanalysis of the Unthought Known*. London: Free Association Books.

——— (1989). *Forces of Destiny: Psychoanalysis and the Human Idiom*. London: Free Association Books.

Bowlby, J. (1988). *A Secure Base: Parent–child Attachment and Healthy Human Development*. New York: Basic Books.

Bowles, D. D. (1988). Development of an ethnic self-concept among blacks. In *Ethnicity and Race: Critical Concepts in Social Work,* ed. C. Jacobs and D. D. Bowles, pp. 103–113. Silver Spring, MD: National Association of Social Workers.

Brazelton, T. B. (1982). Joint regulation of neonate–parent behavior. In *Social Interchange in Infancy*, ed. E. Tronick. Baltimore, MD: University Park Press.

Brown, L. J. (1981). The therapeutic milieu in the treatment of patients with borderline personality disorders. *Bulletin of the Menninger Clinic* 45:377–394.

Carter, B., and McGoldrick, M., eds. (1989). *The Changing Family Life Cycle*. Boston: Allyn & Bacon.

Casement, P. (1991). *Learning from the Patient*. New York: Guilford.

Caudill, W., and Weinstein, H. (1969). Maternal care and infant behavior in Japan and America. *Psychiatry* 32:12– 43.

Chescheir, M. W. (1985). Some implications of Winnicott's concepts for clinical practice. *Clinical Social Work Journal* 13:218–233.

Chescheir, M. W., and Schulz, K. M. (1989). The development of a capacity for concern in antisocial children: Winnicott's concept of human relatedness. *Clinical Social Work Journal* 17:24–39.

Clancier, A., and Kalmanovitch, J. (1987). *Winnicott and Paradox: From Birth to Creation*. New York: Tavistock.

Comstock, C. D. (1981). Inanimate object attachments of elderly nursing home residents. *Smith College Studies in Social Work* 51:192–215.

Davis, M., and Wallbridge, D. (1981). *Boundary and Space: An Introduction to the Work of D. W. Winnicott*. New York: Brunner/Mazel.

Dean, R. G. (1989). Ways of knowing in clinical practice. *Clinical Social Work Journal* 17:116–127.

Dean, R. G. (1993). Constructivism: an approach to clinical practice. *Smith College Studies in Social Work* 63:127–146.

DeJonghe, F., Rijnierse, P., and Janssen, R. (1992). The role of support in psychoanalysis. *Journal of the American Psychoanalytic Association* 40:475–499.

Deri, S. (1984). *Symbolization and Creativity*. New York: International Universities Press.

Dockar-Drysdale, B. (1991). *The Provision of Primary Experience: Winnicottian Work with Children and Adolescents*. Northvale, NJ: Jason Aronson.

Downey, T. W. (1978). Transitional phenomena in the analysis of early adolescent males. *Psychoanalytic Study of the Child* 33:19–46. New Haven, CT: Yale University Press.

Eigen, M. (1989). Aspects of omniscience. In *The Facilitating Environment: Clinical Applications of Winnicott's Theory*, eds. M. G. Fromm and B. L. Smith, pp. 604–628. Madison, CT: International Universities Press.

Emde, R. (1981). Changing models of infancy and the nature of early development: remodeling the foundation. *Journal of the American Psychoanalytic Association* 29:179–220.

Fintzy, R. T. (1971). Vicissitudes of the transitional object in a borderline child. *International Journal of Psycho-Analysis* 52:107–114.

Fisher, S. M. (1975). On the development of the capacity to use transitional objects. *Journal of the American Academy of Child Psychiatry* 14:114–124.

Fox, R. P. (1977). Transitional phenomena in the treatment of a psychotic adolescent. *International Journal of Psychoanalytic Psychotherapy* 6:147–164.

Frankenberg, F. R. (1984). Hoarding in anorexia nervosa. *British Journal of Medical Psychology* 57:57–60.

Freud, S. (1900). The interpretation of dreams. *Standard Edition* 4/5:xxiii– 627.

——— (1914). Remembering, repeating, and working through. *Standard Edition* 12:143–153.

——— (1920). Beyond the pleasure principle. *Standard Edition* 18:3–64.

Fromm, M. G. (1989). Winnicott's work in relation to classical psychoanalysis and ego psychology. In *The Facilitating*

Environment: Clinical Applications of Winnicott's Theory, ed. M. G. Fromm and B. L. Smith, pp. 3–26. Madison, CT: International Universities Press.

Fromm, M. G., and Smith, B. L. (1989). *The Facilitating Environment: Clinical Applications of Winnicott's Theory.* Madison, CT: International Universities Press.

Gaddini, R. (1978). Transitional object origins and the psychosomatic symptom. In *Between Reality and Fantasy: Transitional Objects and Phenomena,* ed. S. A. Grolnick and L. Barkin, pp. 109–132. Northvale, NJ: Jason Aronson.

Gehrie, M. J. (1979). Culture and internal representation. *Psychiatry* 42:165–170.

Giovacchini, P. L., ed. (1990). *Tactics and Techniques in Psychoanalytic Therapy III: The Implications of Winnicott's Contributions.* Northvale, NJ: Jason Aronson.

Goldman, D. (1993a). *In One's Bones: The Clinical Genius of Winnicott.* Northvale, NJ: Jason Aronson.

––––– (1993b). *In Search of the Real: The Origins and Originality of D. W. Winnicott.* Northvale, NJ: Jason Aronson.

Goldstein, E. G. (1984). *Ego Psychology and Social Work Practice.* New York: Free Press.

Gorman, J. (1993). Postmodernism and the conduct of inquiry in social work. *Affilia* 8:247–264.

Green, A. (1978). Potential space in psychoanalysis: the object in the setting. In *Between Reality and Fantasy: Transitional Objects and Phenomena,* ed. S. A. Grolnick and L. Barkin, pp. 169–189. New York: Jason Aronson.

Greenberg, J. R., and Mitchell, S. A. (1983). *Object Relations in Psychoanalytic Theory.* Cambridge, MA: Harvard University Press.

Greenberg, M., and Morris, N. (1974). Engrossment: the newborn's impact upon the father. *American Journal of Orthopsychiatry* 44:520–531.

Greenspan, S. J. (1977). The oedipal-pre-oedipal dilemma: a reformulation according to object relations theory. *International Review of Psycho-Analysis* 4:381–391.

Grolnick, S. A. (1990). *The Work and Play of Winnicott.* Northvale, NJ: Jason Aronson.

Grolnick, S. A., and Barkin, L., eds. (1978). *Between Reality and*

Fantasy: Transitional Objects and Phenomena. Northvale, NJ: Jason Aronson.

Grosskurth, P. (1986). *Melanie Klein: Her World and Her Work*. New York: Knopf.

Gunderson, J. G. (1978). Defining the therapeutic process in psychiatric milieus. *Psychiatry* 41:327–335.

Guntrip, H. (1975). My experience of analysis with Fairbairn & Winnicott (how complete a result does psycho-analytic therapy achieve?). *International Review of Psycho-Analysis* 2:145–156.

Hanna, E. A. (1993). The implications of shifting perspectives in countertransference on the therapeutic action of clinical social work, part I: the classical and early-totalist position. *Journal of Analytic Social Work* 1(3):25–52.

Hartmann, H. (1939). *Ego Psychology and the Problem of Adaptation*. New York: International Universities Press.

Hawkins, P., and Shohet, R. (1989). *Supervision in the Helping Professions*. Philadelphia: Open University Press.

Hegel, G. W. F. (1807). *Phenomenology of Spirit*, trans. A. V. Miller. London: Oxford University Press, 1977.

Horner, A. J. (1979). *Object Relations and the Developing Ego in Therapy*. Northvale, NJ: Jason Aronson.

Horton, P. C., Gewirtz, H., and Kreutter, K. J., eds. (1988). *The Solace Paradigm: An Eclectic Search for Psychological Immunity*. Madison, CT: International Universities Press.

Hughes, J. M. (1989). *Reshaping the Psychoanalytic Domain: The Work of Melanie Klein, W. R. D. Fairbairn, and D. W. Winnicott*. Berkeley and Los Angeles, CA: University of California Press.

Kagan, J. (1984). *The Nature of the Child*. New York: Basic Books.

Kahne, M. J. (1967). On the persistence of transitional phenomena into adult life. *International Journal of Psycho-Analysis* 48:247–258.

Kanter, J. (1990). Community-based management of psychotic clients: the contributions of D. W. and Clare Winnicott. *Clinical Social Work Journal* 18:23–41.

Kaplan, L. J. (1987). The interpersonal world of the infant: a symposium. *Contemporary Psychoanalysis* 23:27–44.

Kestenberg, J. S. (1978). Transsensus-outgoingness and Winnicott's intermediate zone. In *Between Reality and Fantasy:*

Transitional Objects and Phenomena, ed. S. A. Grolnick and L. Barkin, pp. 61–73. Northvale, NJ: Jason Aronson.

Khan, M. M. (1975). Introduction. In *Through Paediatrics to Psycho-Analysis*, D. W. Winnicott, pp. xi–1. New York: Basic Books.

Klein, M. (1975). *Envy and Gratitude and Other Works, 1946–1963.* New York: Delacorte.

Kohut, H. (1971). *The Analysis of the Self.* New York: International Universities Press.

——— (1977). *The Restoration of the Self.* New York: International Universities Press.

Lipscomb, J., and Wander, B., producers (1986). Life's first feelings. *NOVA.* Boston: WGBH-TV.

Little, M. I. (1985). Winnicott working in areas where psychotic anxieties predominate: a personal record. *Free Associations* 3:9– 42.

——— (1990). *Psychotic Anxieties and Containment: A Personal Record of an Analysis with Winnicott.* Northvale, NJ: Jason Aronson.

Mackey, R. A. (1985). *Ego Psychology and Clinical Practice.* New York: Gardner Press.

Mahler, M., and McDevitt, J. B. (1980). The separation-individuation process and identity formation. In *The Course of Life: Psychoanalytic Contributions Towards Understanding Personality Development, vol. 2: Infancy and Early Childhood*, ed. S. Greenspan and G. H. Pollack, pp. 19–35. Washington, DC: National Institute of Mental Health.

Mahler, M., Pine, F., and Bergman, A. (1975). *The Psychological Birth of the Human Infant.* New York: Basic Books.

Martinez, C. (1988). Mexican-Americans. In *Clinical Guidelines in Cross-cultural Mental Health*, ed. L. Comas-Diaz and E. E. H. Griffith, pp. 182–203. New York: John Wiley & Sons.

McDonald, M. (1970). *Not By the Color of Their Skin.* New York: International Universities Press.

McGee, J. J., Menolascino, F. J., Hobbs, D. C., and Menousek, P. E. (1987). *Gentle Teaching: A Non-aversive Approach to Helping Persons with Mental Retardation.* New York: Human Sciences Press.

Meyer, W. (1993). In defense of long-term treatment: on the vanishing holding environment. *Social Work* 38:571–578.

Milner, M. (1978). D. W. Winnicott and the two-way journey. In *Between Reality and Fantasy: Transitional Objects and Phenomena*, ed. S. A. Grolnick and L. Barkin, pp. 15–34. Northvale, NJ: Jason Aronson.

Modell, A. H. (1976). "The holding environment" and the therapeutic action of psychoanalysis. *Journal of the American Psychoanalytic Association* 24:285–307.

Ogden, T. H. (1976). Psychological unevenness in the academically successful student. *International Journal of Psychoanalytic Psychotherapy* 5:437–447.

——— (1989). Playing, dreaming, and interpreting experience: comments on potential space. In *The Facilitating Environment: Clinical Applications of Winnicott's Theory*, ed. M. G. Fromm and B. L. Smith, pp. 255–278. Madison, CT: International Universities Press.

——— (1990). *The Matrix of the Mind: Object Relations and the Psychoanalytic Dialogue*. Northvale, NJ: Jason Aronson.

Panel. (1968). Aspects of culture in psychoanalytic theory and practice. *Journal of the American Psychoanalytic Association* 16:651–670.

Parens, H. (1979). *The Development of Aggression in Early Childhood*. Northvale, NJ: Jason Aronson.

Phillips, A. (1988). *Winnicott*. Cambridge, MA: Harvard University Press.

Pinderhughes, E., Kirkpatrick, W., Panasevich, K., et al. (1979). *The effect of ethnicity upon the psychological task of separation-individuation: a comparison of four ethnic groups*. Paper presented at the Annual Meeting of the American Orthopsychiatric Association, Washington, DC, March/April.

Pine, F. (1985). *Developmental Theory and Clinical Process*. New Haven, CT: Yale University Press.

——— (1988). The four psychologies of psychoanalysis and their place in clinical work. *Journal of the American Psychoanalytic Association* 36:571–596.

——— (1990). *Drive, Ego, Object, and Self: A Synthesis for Clinical Work*. New York: Basic Books.

Polanyi, M. (1962). *Personal Knowledge: Towards a Post-critical Philosophy*. Chicago: University of Chicago Press.

Popple, P. R. (1983). Contexts of practice. In *Handbook of Clinical*

Social Work, ed. A. Rosenblatt and D. Waldfogel, pp. 70–96. San Francisco: Jossey-Bass.

Provence, S., and Ritvo, S. (1961). Effects of deprivation on institutionalized infants: disturbances in development of relationships to inanimate objects. *The Psychoanalytic Study of the Child* 16:189–205. New York: International Universities Press.

Pruett, K. D. (1983). Infants of primary nurturing fathers. *The Psychoanalytic Study of the Child* 38:257–277. New Haven, CT: Yale University Press.

Ramos-McKay, J. M., Comas-Diaz, L., and Rivera, L. A. (1988). Puerto Ricans. In *Clinical Guidelines in Cross-cultural Mental Health*, ed. L. Comas-Diaz and E. E. H. Griffith, pp. 204–232. New York: John Wiley & Sons.

Richardson, L. (1994). Writing: a method of inquiry. In *Handbook of Qualitative Research*, ed. N. K. Denzin and Y. S. Lincoln, pp. 516–529. Thousand Oaks, CA: Sage.

Ritvo, S. (1971). Late adolescence: developmental and clinical considerations. *The Psychoanalytic Study of the Child* 26:241–263. New Haven, CT: Yale University Press.

Rodman, F. R. (1987). *The Spontaneous Gesture: Selected Letters of D. W. Winnicott*. Cambridge, MA: Harvard University Press.

Ross, J. M. (1993). The clinical relevance of the contributions of Winnicott. *Journal of the American Psychoanalytic Association* 41:219–235.

Ross, M. H. (in press). Psychocultural interpretation theory and peacemaking in ethnic conflicts. *Political Psychology.*

Rudnytsky, P. L. (1991). *The Psychoanalytic Vocation: Rank, Winnicott, and the Legacy of Freud*. New Haven, CT: Yale University Press.

Saari, C. (1986). *Clinical Social Work Treatment: How Does It Work?* New York: Gardner Press.

—— (1988). Interpretation: event or process? *Clinical Social Work Journal* 16:378–390.

—— (1990). The process of learning in clinical social work. *Smith College Studies in Social Work* 60:35–49.

—— (1991). *The Creation of Meaning in Clinical Social Work*. New York: Guilford.

—— (1994). Empathy in clinical social work: playing in transcontextual space. *Journal of Analytic Social Work* 2:25–42.

Sacksteder, J. L. (1989). Psychosomatic dissociation and false self development in anorexia nervosa. In *The Facilitating Environment: Clinical Applications of Winnicott's Theory*, ed. M. G. Fromm and B. L. Smith, pp. 365–393. Madison, CT: International Universities Press.

Saleebey, D. (1989). The estrangement of knowing and doing: professions in crisis. *Social Casework* 70:556–563.

——— (1994). Culture, theory, and narrative: the intersection of meanings in practice. *Social Work* 39:351–359.

Sanville, J. (1991). *The Playground of Psychoanalytic Therapy*. Hillsdale, NJ: Analytic Press.

Schön, D. A. (1983). *The Reflective Practitioner: How Professionals Think in Action*. New York: Basic Books.

——— (1987). *Educating the Reflective Practitioner*. San Francisco: Jossey-Bass.

Shafii, M. (1973). Adaptive and therapeutic aspects of meditation. *International Journal of Psychoanalytic Psychotherapy* 2:364–382.

Shor, J., and Sanville, J. (1978). *Illusion in Loving: A Psychoanalytic Approach to the Evolution of Intimacy and Autonomy*. Los Angeles: Double Helix Press.

Smith, B. L. (1989). Of many minds: a contribution on the dynamics of multiple personality. In *The Facilitating Environment: Clinical Applications of Winnicott's Theory*, ed. M. G. Fromm and B. L. Smith, pp. 424–458. Madison, CT: International Universities Press.

Spence, D. P. (1982). *Narrative Truth and Historical Truth*. New York: W. W. Norton.

Speers, R. W., and Morter, D. C. (1980). Overindividuation and underseparation in the pseudomature child. In *Rapprochement: The Critical Subphase of Separation-Individuation*, ed. R. L. Lax, S. Bach, and J. A. Burland, pp. 457–478. Northvale, NJ: Jason Aronson.

Spitz, R. A. (1963). In *Dialogues from Infancy*, ed. R. N. Emde. New York: International Universities Press, 1983.

Stack, C. (1975). *All Our Kin*. New York: Harper & Row.

Stamm, I. (1985). The hospital as a "holding environment." *International Journal of Therapeutic Communities* 6:219–229.

Stechler, G., and Halton, A. (1987). The emergence of assertion and aggression during infancy: a psychoanalytic systems approach. *Journal of the American Psychoanalytic Association* 35:821–838.

Stern, D. N. (1985). *The Interpersonal World of the Infant*. New York: Basic Books.

Sugarman, A. (1984). Deanimated transitional phenomena in paranoid conditions: the "influencing machine" revisited. *Bulletin of the Menninger Clinic* 48:418–426.

Sugarman, A., and Kurash, C. (1982). The body as a transitional object in bulimia. *International Journal of Eating Disorders* 1:312–322.

Sutherland, J. D. (1980). The British object relations theorists: Balint, Winnicott, Fairbairn, Guntrip. *Journal of the American Psychoanalytic Association* 28:829–860.

Tolpin, M. (1971). On the beginnings of a cohesive self: an application of the concept of transmuting internalization to the study of the transitional object and signal anxiety. *Psychoanalytic Study of the Child* 26:316–353. New Haven, CT: Yale University Press.

Volkan, V. D. (1973). Transitional fantasies in the analysis of a narcissistic personality. *Journal of the American Psychoanalytic Association* 21:351–376.

——— (1988). *The Need to Have Enemies and Allies: From Clinical Practice to International Relationships*. Northvale, NJ: Jason Aronson.

Weil, A. P. (1970). The basic core. *Psychoanalytic Study of the Child* 25:443–460. New York: International Universities Press.

Werner, H., and Kaplan, B. (1963). *Symbol Formation*. New York: John Wiley & Sons.

Williams, M. (1975). *The Velveteen Rabbit*. New York: Avon.

Winnicott, C. (1989). D. W. W.: a reflection. In *Psycho-Analytic Explorations: D. W. Winnicott*, ed. C. Winnicott, R. Shepherd, and M. Davis, pp. 1–18. Cambridge, MA: Harvard University Press.

Winnicott, C., Shepherd, R., and Davis, M., eds. (1989). *Psychoanalytic Explorations: D. W. Winnicott*. Cambridge, MA: Harvard University Press.

Winnicott, D. W. (1941). The observation of infants in a set situation. In *Through Paediatrics to Psycho-Analysis*, pp. 52–69. New York: Basic Books, 1975.

—— (1945). Primitive emotional development. In *Through Paediatrics to Psycho-Analysis*, pp. 145–156. New York: Basic Books, 1975.

—— (1947). Hate in the countertransference. In *Through Paediatrics to Psycho-Analysis*, pp. 194–203. New York: Basic Books, 1975.

—— (1949). Mind and its relation to psyche-soma. In *Through Paediatrics to Psycho-Analysis*, pp. 243–254. New York: Basic Books, 1975.

—— (1950). Aggression in relation to emotional development. In *Through Paediatrics to Psycho-Analysis*, pp. 204–218. New York: Basic Books, 1975.

—— (1952). Anxiety associated with insecurity. In *Through Paediatrics to Psycho-Analysis*, pp. 97–100. New York: Basic Books, 1975.

—— (1953). Transitional objects and transitional phenomena: a study of the first not-me possession. *International Journal of Psycho-Analysis* 34:89–97.

—— (1954). Metapsychological and clinical aspects of regression within the psycho-analytical set-up. In *Through Paediatrics to Psycho-Analysis*, pp. 278–294. New York: Basic Books, 1975.

—— (1954–1955). The depressive position in normal emotional development. In *Through Paediatrics to Psycho-Analysis*, pp. 262–277. New York: Basic Books, 1975.

—— (1955–1956). Clinical varieties of transference. In *Through Paediatrics to Psycho-Analysis*, pp. 295–299. New York: Basic Books, 1975.

—— (1956a). Primary maternal preoccupation. In *Through Paediatrics to Psycho-Anlaysis*, pp. 300–305. New York: Basic Books, 1975.

—— (1956b). The antisocial tendency. In *Through Paediatrics to Psycho-Analysis*, pp. 306–315. New York: Basic Books, 1975.

—— (1957). Integrative and disruptive factors in family life. In *The Family and Individual Development*, pp. 40–49. London: Routledge, 1989.

———— (1958). The capacity to be alone. In *The Maturational Processes and the Facilitating Environment*, pp. 29–36. Madison, CT: International Universities Press, 1965.

———— (1959–1964). Classification: is there a psycho-analytic contribution to psychiatric classification? In *The Maturational Processes and the Facilitating Environment*, pp. 124–139. Madison, CT: International Universities Press, 1965.

———— (1960a). Counter-transference. In *The Maturational Processes and the Facilitating Environment*, pp. 158–165. Madison, CT: International Universities Press, 1965.

———— (1960b). Ego distortion in terms of true and false self. In *The Maturational Processes and the Facilitating Environment*, pp. 140–152. Madison, CT: International Universities Press, 1965.

———— (1960c). String: a technique of communication. In *The Maturational Processes and the Facilitating Environment*, pp. 153–157. Madison, CT: International Universities Press, 1965.

———— (1960d). The theory of the parent–infant relationship. In *The Maturational Processes and the Facilitating Environment*, pp. 37–55. Madison, CT: International Universities Press, 1965.

———— (1961). Varieties of psychotherapy. In *Home Is Where We Start From: Essays by a Psychoanalyst*, pp. 101–111. New York: W. W. Norton, 1986.

———— (1962a). Ego integration in child development. In *The Maturational Processes and the Facilitating Environment*, pp. 56–63. Madison, CT: International Universities Press, 1965.

———— (1962b). The aims of psycho-analytical treatment. In *The Maturational Processes and the Facilitating Environment*, pp. 166–170. Madison, CT: International Universities Press, 1965.

———— (1962c). Providing for the child in health and in crisis. In *The Maturational Processes and the Facilitating Environment*, pp. 64–72. Madison, CT: International Universities Press, 1965.

———— (1963a). Communicating and not communicating leading

to a study of certain opposites. In *The Maturational Processes and the Facilitating Environment*, pp. 179–192. Madison, CT: International Universities Press, 1965.

———— (1963b). From dependence towards independence in the development of the individual. In *The Maturational Processes and the Facilitating Environment*, pp. 83–92. Madison, CT: International Universities Press, 1965.

———— (1963c). Psychotherapy of character disorders. In *The Maturational Processes and the Facilitating Environment*, pp. 203–216. Madison, CT: International Universities Press, 1965.

———— (1963d). The development of the capacity for concern. In *The Maturational Processes and the Facilitating Environment*, pp. 73–82. Madison, CT: International Universities Press, 1965.

———— (1963e). The mentally ill in your caseload. In *The Maturational Processes and the Facilitating Environment*, pp. 217–229. Madison, CT: International Universities Press, 1965.

———— (1963f). The value of depression. In *Home Is Where We Start From: Essays by a Psychoanalyst*, pp. 71–79. New York: W. W. Norton, 1986.

———— (1965a). *The Family and Individual Development*. London: Tavistock.

———— (1965b). The price of disregarding psychoanalytic research. In *Home Is Where We Start From: Essays by a Psychoanalyst*, pp. 172–182. New York: W. W. Norton, 1986.

———— (1966). The child in the family group. In *Home Is Where We Start From: Essays by a Psychoanalyst*, pp. 128–141. New York: W. W. Norton, 1986.

———— (1967a). Delinquency as a sign of hope. In *Home Is Where We Start From: Essays by a Psychoanalyst*, pp. 90–100. New York: W. W. Norton, 1986.

———— (1967b). The concept of the healthy individual. In *Home Is Where We Start From: Essays by a Psychoanalyst*, pp. 20–38. New York: W. W. Norton., 1986.

———— (1968a). Adolescent immaturity. In *Home Is Where We Start From: Essays by a Psychoanalyst*, pp. 150–166. New York: W. W. Norton, 1986.

———— (1968b). Communication between infant and mother, and mother and infant, compared and contrasted. In *Babies and*

Their Mothers, pp. 89–103. Reading, MA: Addison-Wesley, 1988.

—— (1969). Behavior therapy. In *Psycho-Analytic Explorations: D. W. Winnicott,* ed. C. Winnicott, R. Shepherd, and M. Davis, pp. 558–560. Cambridge, MA: Harvard University Press, 1989.

—— (1970a). Cure. In *Home Is Where We Start From: Essays by a Psychoanalyst,* pp. 112–120. New York: W. W. Norton, 1986.

—— (1970b). Residential care as therapy. In *Deprivation and Delinquency,* ed. C. Winnicott, R. Shepherd, and M. Davis, pp. 220–228. New York: Tavistock, 1984.

—— (1970c). The mother–infant experience of mutuality. In *Parenthood: Its Psychology and Psychopathology,* ed. E. J. Anthony and T. Benedek, pp. 245–256. Boston: Little, Brown.

—— (1971a). Mirror-role of mother and family in child development. In *Playing and Reality,* pp. 111–118. London: Tavistock.

—— (1971b). Playing: A theoretical statement. In *Playing and Reality,* pp. 38–52. London: Tavistock.

—— (1971c). Playing: creative activity and the search for the self. In *Playing and Reality,* pp. 53–64. London: Tavistock.

—— (1971d). The location of cultural experience. In *Playing and Reality,* pp. 95–103. London: Tavistock.

—— (1971e). The use of an object and relating through identifications. In *Playing and Reality,* pp. 86–94. London: Tavistock.

—— (1971f). *Therapeutic Consultations in Child Psychiatry.* London: Hogarth.

—— (1974). Fear of breakdown. *International Review of Psycho-Analysis* 1:103–107.

—— (1977). *The Piggle: An Account of the Psychoanalytic Treatment of a Little Girl.* New York: International Universities Press.

—— (1986a). *Holding and Interpretation: Fragment of an Analysis.* New York: Hogarth.

—— (1986b). *Home Is Where We Start From: Essays by a Psychoanalyst.* New York: W. W. Norton.

—— (1988a). *Babies and their Mothers.* Reading, MA: Addison-Wesley.

—— (1988b). *Human Nature.* New York: Schocken Books.

—— (1993). *Talking to Parents.* Reading, MA: Addison-Wesley.

Wolff, P. (1959). Observations on newborn infants. *Psychosomatic Medicine* 2:110–118.

Wolman, T. (1991). Mahler and Winnicott: some parallels in their lives and work. In *Beyond the Symbiotic Orbit. Advances in Separation-Individuation Theory: Essays in Honor of Selma Kramer,* ed. S. Akhtar and H. Parens, pp. 35–60. Hillsdale, NJ: Analytic Press.

Yerushalmi, H. (1992). Psychoanalytic supervision and the need to be alone. *Psychotherapy* 29:262–268.

Zeanah, C. H., Anders, T. F., Seifer, R., and Stern, D. N. (1989). Implications of research on infant development for psychodynamic theory and practice. *Journal of the American Academy of Child and Adolescent Psychiatry* 28:657–668.

Zerbe, D. H. (1990). The therapist at play and the patient who begins to play. *Clinical Social Work Journal* 18:9–22.

CREDITS

The authors gratefully acknowledge permission to quote from the following sources:

Excerpts from *The Maturational Processes and the Facilitating Environment*, by D. W. Winnicott. Copyright © 1965 by International Universities Press and The Hogarth Press, London (part of Random House UK). Reproduced by permission of Mark Paterson and Associates on behalf of the publishers and The Winnicott Trust.

Excerpts from "Winnicott and Clinical Social Work: A Facilitating Partnership," by Jeffrey S. Applegate in *Child and Adolescent Social Work*, vol. 10, no. 1, pp. 3–19. Copyright © 1993 by Plenum Publishing Corporation.

Excerpts from "Transitional Phenomena in Adolescence: Tools for Negotiating the Second Individuation," by Jeffrey

INDEX

Internalization, developmental
theory, 30
Interpersonal relationships. *See
also* Ego relatedness
aggression and, 50
holding environment,
assessment of, 101–103
infant development and, 8–9
interdependence and, 55–58
Interpretation
interventions, for disturbed
development, 78–79
suspicion of, 21
Intersubjectivity, infant
development and, 41
Intervention
antisocial tendency, object
relating/use, 193–194
for disturbed development,
76–80
ego relatedness, 129–153
capacity to be alone,
difficulties with, 149–
153
drive and impulse
difficulties, 148–149
generally, 129–130
involuntary clients, 136–
147
primary attachment
difficulties, 130–136
holding environment, 109–
119
for disturbed development,
78–79
generally, 109
handling, 112–113
holding, 109–112
object presentation, 113–
119
potential space and, 234
transitional process, 165–176

Intrapsychic dimension,
holding environment,
assessment of, 103–107
Involuntary clients, ego
relatedness, assessment and
intervention, 136–147
Involvement, holding
environment intervention,
110

Kahne, M. J., 174
Kalmanovitch, J., 11, 15
Kanter, J., 12, 16, 87
Kaplan, B., 102, 146, 237
Kestenberg, J. S., 125
Khan, M. M., 8, 17, 20, 21, 258
Klein, M., 17, 22, 50, 52, 66, 250
Kohut, H., 34, 67, 206
Kurash, C., 67, 169

Language acquisition, object
relating/object use, 55
Libido, developmental theory
and, 39–40
Lipscomb, J., 126
Little, M. I., 20, 86

Mackey, R. A., 7
Mahler, M., 38, 43, 45, 51, 53,
55, 67, 206, 240
Managed care, 257–260
Manic defense, disturbed
development, holding
environment, 66
Marijuana, transitional process,
173–174
Martinez, C., 236
Master, object relating/use and,
241
Mastery
aggression and, 49
dependency and, 15